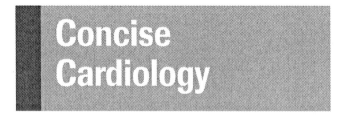

Concise Cardiology

An Evidence-Based Handbook

Concise Cardiology

An Evidence-Based Handbook

EDITOR
David V. Daniels, MD
Fellow in Cardiovascular Medicine
Fellow in Critical Care Medicine
Stanford University Medical Center
Stanford, California

ASSOCIATE EDITORS
Stanley G. Rockson, MD
Chief of Consultative Cardiology
Stanford University Medical Center
Stanford, California

Randall Vagelos, MD
Professor of Medicine/Medical Director, CCU
Cardiovascular Medicine
Stanford University Medical Center
Stanford, California

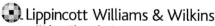
. Lippincott Williams & Wilkins
a Wolters Kluwer business
Philadelphia · Baltimore · New York · London
Buenos Aires · Hong Kong · Sydney · Tokyo

Acquisitions Editor: Frances R. DeStefano
Managing Editor: Chris Potash
Project Manager: Rosanne Hallowell
Manufacturing Manager: Kathleen Brown
Marketing Manager: Kimberly Schonberger
Design Coordinator: Teresa Mallon
Cover Designer: Lou Fuiano
Production Services: Elm Street Publishing Services

530 Walnut Street
Philadelphia, PA 19106
LWW.com

Printed in China

Library of Congress Cataloging-in-Publication Data
Concise cardiology : an evidence-based handbook / editor, David V. Daniels; associate editors, Stanley G. Rockson, Randall Vagelos.
    p.   ;   cm.
Includes bibliographical references and index.
ISBN 978-0-7817-8509-9
1. Cardiology—Handbooks, manuals, etc.   2. Heart—Diseases—Handbooks, manuals, etc.   I. Daniels, David V.   II. Rockson, Stanley G.   III. Vagelos, Randall.
[DNLM: 1. Heart Diseases—Handbooks.   2. Diagnostic Techniques, Cardiovascular—Handbooks.   3. Evidence-Based Medicine—Handbooks.
WG 39 C755 2008]
RC669.15C66 2008
616.1'2—dc22

                                                                    2008009965

Care has been taken to confirm the accuracy of the information presented and to describe generally accepted practices. However, the authors, editors, and publisher are not responsible for errors or omissions or for any consequences from application of the information in this book and make no warranty, expressed or implied, with respect to the currency, completeness, or accuracy of the contents of the publication. Application of this information in a particular situation remains the professional responsibility of the practitioner.

The authors, editors, and publisher have exerted every effort to ensure that drug selection and dosage set forth in this text are in accordance with current recommendations and practice at the time of publication. However, in view of ongoing research, changes in government regulations, and the constant flow of information relating to drug therapy and drug reactions, the reader is urged to check the package insert for each drug for any change in indications and dosage and for added warnings and precautions. This is particularly important when the recommended agent is a new or infrequently employed drug.

Some drugs and medical devices presented in this publication have Food and Drug Administration (FDA) clearance for limited use in restricted research settings. It is the responsibility of health care providers to ascertain the FDA status of each drug or device planned for use in their clinical practice.

The publishers have made every effort to trace copyright holders for borrowed material. If they have inadvertently overlooked any, they will be pleased to make the necessary arrangements at the first opportunity.

To purchase additional copies of this book, call our customer service department at (800) 638-3030 or fax orders to (301) 223-2320. International customers should call (301) 223-2300.

Visit Lippincott Williams & Wilkins on the Internet at LWW.com. Lippincott Williams & Wilkins customer service representatives are available from 8:30 am to 6 pm, EST.

10 9 8 7 6 5 4 3

First, to Mom and Dad: You are the best parents anyone could ever hope for and you will always be with me. I am forever grateful for the infinite lessons, constant patience, and values you have bestowed upon me. You always had faith in me, often when I was unsure of myself, and I can only aspire to have the same courage and compassion with my own children someday.

My sister Ana, my brother-in law Bart, and my princess Stefanie: We are family forever, and it is one of the only things in this world I am truly sure of. I am blessed with best friends that are closer than many boys are to their own brothers and I hope to never take that for granted.

I want to thank the many great teachers in my life, especially the ones who nurtured a rigorous academic approach tempered with habitual common sense. These are lessons that no textbook can confer.

CONTENTS

CONTRIBUTORS

Amin Al-Ahmad, MD
Assistant Professor of Cardiovascular Medicine
Associate Director, Cardiac Arrythmia Services
Stanford University
Stanford, California

Euan Ashley, MRCP, DPhil
Assistant Professor of Medicine
Cardiovascular Medicine
Stanford University
Stanford, California

Todd J. Brinton, MD
Instructor of Medicine (Cardiology)
Lecturer in Bioengineering
Interventional Cardiology
Stanford, California

Ian Brown, MS, MD
Instructor of Surgery (Emergency Medicine)
Stanford University School of Medicine
Stanford, California

Kamalendu Chatterjee, MB, FRCP, FACC, FCCP, MACP
Ernest Gallo Distinguished Professor of Medicine
Division of Cardiology, Department of Medicine
University of California
San Francisco, California

Clarke G. Daniels, MD
Cardiologist, Internal Medicine
Doctor's Medical Center—San Pablo
San Pablo, California

David V. Daniels, MD
Fellow in Cardiovascular Medicine
Fellow in Critical Care Medicine
Stanford University Medical Center
Stanford, California

Ramona L. Doyle, MD
Associate Professor
Division of Pulmonary/Critical Care Medicine
Department of Medicine
Stanford University
Stanford, California

James V. Freeman, MD, MPH
Fellow in Cardiovascular Medicine
Stanford University
Stanford, California

Anurag Gupta, MD
Electrophysiology Fellow
Department of Medicine, Division of Cardiology
Stanford University Hospital
Stanford, California

François Haddad, MD
Clinical Instructor of Medicine, Division of Cardiovascular Medicine
Attending Cardiologist
Heart Failure and Transplant Service
Pulmonary Hypertension Service
Stanford University School of Medicine
Stanford, California

Henry Hsia, MD
Associate Professor, Cardiovascular Medicine
Assistant Director, Arrhythmia Services
Stanford Medical Center
Stanford, California

David Kao, MD
NASA Ames Research Center
Chief Medicine Resident
Stanford University
Stanford, California

Todd L. Kiefer, MD, PhD
Fellow, Cardiovascular Medicine
Duke University Medical Center
Durham, North Carolina

David P. Lee, MD
Director, Cardiac Catheterization and Coronary Internist
Assistant Professor
Stanford University School of Medicine
Stanford, California

Juliana C. Liu, RN, MSN, ANP
Nurse Practitioner
Vera M. Wall Center for Pulmonary Vascular Disease
Pulmonary and Critical Care Medicine
Stanford University
Stanford, California

Fred A. Lopez, MD, FACP
Associate Professor and Vice Chair
Louisiana State University, Department of Medicine
LSU Health Sciences Center
New Orleans, Louisiana

Kelly Matsuda, PharmD
Clinical Pharmacist
(Cardiovascular) Pharmacy
Stanford University Medical Center
Stanford, California

Shriram Nallamshetty, MD
Cardiology Fellow
Department of Medicine, Cardiology Division
Massachusetts General Hospital
Boston, Massachusetts

Michael Pham, MD, MPH
Instructor, Cardiology Division
Stanford University School of Medicine
Medical Director, Heart Failure and Transplant Program
VA Palo Alto Healthcare System
Palo Alto, California

Stanley G. Rockson, MD
Chief of Consultative Cardiology
Stanford University Medical Center
Stanford, California

Donald Schreiber, MD, CM
Associate Professor, Surgery (Emergency Medicine)
Attending Physician, Emergency Medicine
Stanford University Hospital
Stanford, California

Randall Vagelos, MD
Professor of Medicine/Medical Director, CCU
Cardiovascular Medicine
Stanford University
Stanford, California

Paul J. Wang
Director, Cardiac Electrophysiology and Arrythmia Service
Professor of Medicine
Stanford University School of Medicine
Stanford, California

Roham T. Zamanian, MD, FCCP
Assistant Professor of Medicine
Division of Pulmonary and Critical Care Medicine
Director, Adult Pulmonary Hypertension Clinical Services
Stanford University School of Medicine
Stanford, California

FOREWORD

To study the phenomenon of disease without books is to sail an uncharted sea, while to study books without patients is not to go to sea at all.

— Sir William Osler

While we recognize the comprehensive nature of classic textbooks like *Braunwald's Heart Disease* and cutting-edge resources like *Up-to-Date*, a void still remains in the cardiology literature. Residents in training, cardiology fellows, and those in practice alike operate in a fast-paced environment where realistically the ability to look something up depends on having a resource that can be consulted in the time it takes the elevator to go from floor 1 to floor 3. Such a resource must be concise and current, and must present the most reasonable clinical approach and the landmark evidence to back it up.

Written as a collaborative effort by residents and fellows in training and experienced attending physicians, *Concise Cardiology: An Evidence-Based Handbook* will serve a niche in our field. It is a truly comprehensive handbook that covers topics from acute coronary syndromes to electrophysiology to valvular heart disease. Each chapter begins with a robust dissection of the clinical problem, starting with relevant historical and physical exam findings to aid in the diagnostic process. Therapies are organized in chart format where appropriate, presenting indications, patient selection, and side effects. Choice of treatment is of course influenced by the best available evidence, and this handbook delivers—not only with a strong base of recommendations from the ACC/AHA but also with a review of "landmark clinical trials," from the historical data to the latest therapies. One of the most unique aspects of our handbook is this easy-to-use, no-nonsense tabular presentation of the landmark evidence that shapes cardiology today. The evidence is pared down to the most critical information clinicians need to make rational treatment decisions, such as level of evidence, patient population studied, intervention, background therapies, outcomes, and number needed to treat. The initial portion of each chapter focuses on management and is targeted primarily toward residents, while the landmark evidence sections will be useful to fellows in training.

Alan Yeung
Professor of Medicine
Division Chief, Cardiology
Stanford University Medical Center

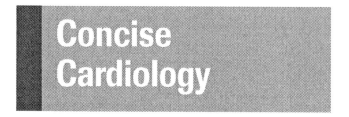

Concise Cardiology

An Evidence-Based Handbook

Physical Examination of the Cardiovascular System

CLARKE G. DANIELS, DAVID V. DANIELS,
AND KAMALENDU CHATTERJEE

BACKGROUND AND APPROACH

An 81-year-old patient presented to the emergency room complaining of weakness and fatigue. His family had noted mild disorientation. Physical exam revealed blood pressure (BP) 113/73, temperature 100°F, and heart rate (HR) 130. The lungs were clear. He was given 2 liters of intravenous normal saline. The chest x-ray subsequently showed pulmonary congestion, and the patient was found to have a cardiomyopathy and markedly reduced ejection fraction.

Doctors at all levels of training and experience make errors in diagnosis. Every doctor has made many mistakes for a variety of reasons; many of these are unavoidable. Failure to recognize heart failure when physical findings are present is not a rare occurrence. I believe this also applies to other common cardiovascular disorders. Did the doctor in this hypothetical narrative know how to evaluate the venous pressure and how to listen for a third heart sound? These are skills that, with practice, can be learned at an early stage of training.

Accordingly, the emphasis in this section will be limited to physical findings that I think a trainee should know in detail in order to evaluate the following diseases. Many findings discussed in a standard textbook of medicine are not covered. The focus will be on physical findings in common diseases and conditions that demand early recognition because of their serious nature, such as the following:

* Congestive heart failure and left ventricular dysfunction
* Acute and chronic pulmonary hypertension
* Complications of myocardial infarction
* Cardiac tamponade

- Mitral aortić (pulmonic) and tricuspid valve disease
- Innocent murmurs
- Dilated and hypertrophic cardiomyopathy
- Atrial septal defect (ASD) and ventricular septal defect (VSD)

HEART SOUNDS

Normal First and Second Heart Sounds

- Intensity of the first heart sound is related to the rapidity of closure of the mitral valve, which is dependent on the left ventricular-left atrial pressure gradient in late diastole, the position of the mitral valve immediately before complete closure, and left ventricular dp/dt.
- The first heart sound is best appreciated at the apical impulse in the left decubitus position.
- Narrow splitting of the S1 representing tricuspid and mitral closure sounds may be heard in normals.
- A2 and P2 refer to the two components of the second heart sound.
- The intensity of the A2 or P2 is related to the pressures against which aortic and pulmonary valves close. Because aortic diastolic pressure is normally significantly higher than the pulmonary artery diastolic pressure, A2 is much louder than the P2 (for abnormal intensity of heart sounds, see Table 1-1).
- Splitting of S2 is usually heard best at the left sternal border in the second and third interspace using the diaphragm of the stethoscope.
- Normally, P2 occurs later than A2 because pulmonary artery "hang out time" is longer than the aortic "hang out time." The pulmonary hang out normally is about 60 msec and that of the aorta is about 20 to 30 msec. The difference between these two hang out times explains why P2 follows A2 and also the differences in normal splitting of the second heart sound. The hang out times are primarily determined by pulmonary artery and aortic compliance, pulmonary and aortic pressures and right and left ventricular stroke volumes.[1]
- During inspiration, P2 is further delayed as a result of further prolongation of the pulmonary artery hang out time due to transient increase in right ventricular stroke volume during inspiration. (Note that decreased impedance decreases ventricular ejection time, and increased impedance prolongs ventricular ejection time. Normal earlier electrical activation of the left ventricle causes a minor contribution for earlier A2, and higher LV dp/dt similarly also contributes, to a rather small extent, to the normal A2-P2 interval.)
- The normal second heart sound is thus usually split with inspiration and single with expiration in children and younger adults. In older adults (over age 50) it is commonly single in all phases of respiration.[2] (for abnormal splitting of heart sounds, see Table 1-2).

TABLE 1-1   Abnormal intensity of heart sounds

	Soft	Loud
S1	• First degree A-V block • Decreased left ventricular contractility • Acute severe aortic insufficiency with premature closure of the mitral valve • Thickening and calcification of the mitral valve resulting in reduced mobility	• Hyperkinetic circulation as in children, hyperthyroidism, anemia, fever, etc. • A short P-R interval • Mitral stenosis when the valve cusps are mobile. This is believed to be as a result of prolongation of diastolic flow providing a large excursion of the valve leaflets and a loud sound as they strike the valve ring • Variability of intensity of S1 occurs when the rhythm is *irregular* due to variations in excursion of the mitral valve • Variability of intensity of S1, in the presence of *regular* rhythm, suggests the presence of A-V dissociation as in complete heart block or ventricular tachycardia
S2	• A soft P2 in comparison to A2 may be heard in valvular pulmonary stenosis due to valve deformity and decreased pulmonary artery diastolic pressure • Similarly, A2 is often soft in severe valvular aortic stenosis because of relative reduction of aortic diastolic pressure • Since this latter condition occurs frequently in older adults where the second heart sound is often single, a single soft second heart sound may be heard or the second heart sound may be absent • In the elderly patients with aortic stenosis with history of arterial hypertension, the intensity of A2 may be preserved or even louder	• A loud A2 may be heard in systemic hypertension or in hyperkinetic states such as thyrotoxicosis or aortic regurgitation • A P2 equal in loudness or louder than A2 is heard in pulmonary hypertension, either chronic such as in primary pulmonary hypertension, or acute as in pulmonary embolism

TABLE 1-2 Abnormal splitting of heart sounds

Persistent	Fixed	Paradoxical
Wide on expiration and wider on inspiration	*No (or only slight) phasic variation in the splitting during the respiratory cycle in all positions*	*During inspiration, P2 becomes delayed and occurs simultaneously with A2 or after A2. This results in splitting in expiration (A2 follows P2) and a single S2 in inspiration (A2 and P2 occur simultaneously). This is referred to as paradoxical splitting*
S1 • Right bundle branch block • Premature ventricular complexes (PVCs) • Ventricular tachycardia • Atrial septal defects • Ebstein's anomaly[3]		

4

S2

* Right bundle branch block
* Type A Wolff-Parkinson-White syndrome presumably as a result of delayed activation of the right ventricle
* Left ventricular pacing as during biventricular pacing
* In valvular pulmonary artery stenosis the second heart sound is widely split and the degree of splitting is directly related to the severity of the right ventricular out-flow obstruction. The splitting of the second heart sound is not usually fixed until the right ventricular stroke volume is also fixed

* In atrial septal defect, there is increased pulmonary vascular capacitance and increased pulmonary blood flow as a result of the shunt. This results in a delayed P2 and wide splitting of the second heart sound. Inspiration does not further increase pulmonary blood flow and there is redistribution of pulmonary and systemic blood flow and hence the duration of splitting is *relatively fixed*

* Left bundle branch block and hence delayed activation of the left ventricle, A2 may be delayed and occur after P2 in expiration
* Other causes of paradoxical splitting of S2 include left ventricular outflow tract obstruction such as hypertrophic obstructive cardiomyopathy and severe aortic valvular stenosis. Right ventricular PVCs, and right ventricular pacing may also cause paradoxical splitting due to electrical delay in left ventricular activation, significant aortic regurgitation due to the selective increase in left ventricular stroke volume[1]

- A2 is louder than P2 when listening in the second left interspace in 70% of normal subjects under age 20, and it is always louder than P2 in subjects over age 20.[2]
- "Normal children, young adults, and trained athletes, may have *persistent* splitting of S2 when examined supine, which disappears when they sit or stand owing to decreased venous return. By contrast, S2 remains audibly split during expiration in pathologic conditions, even when the patient is examined sitting or standing."[3]

The Third Heart Sound (S3 or Ventricular Gallop)

- This sound may normally be heard in children and young adults, pregnant women, and trained athletes.
- In the context of other evidence of heart disease, an S3 correlates with elevated ventricular end diastolic pressure and also to elevated B-type natriuretic peptide (BNP) in patients with systolic heart failure.
- It is best timed by focusing on the *second* heart sound followed by a brief *interval* after S2, followed by S3. The interval is longer than the A2-P2 interval and longer than the S2 opening snap interval. It may be faint and best heard when focusing on the instant when it is expected; that is to say, "tuning in."[3]
- It is a low-frequency sound, best heard with soft application of the bell over the apical impulse, with the patient lying on the left side. An outward movement of the apex may be noted that is synchronous with the S3 (visible and audible). This is further confirmation that the sound is an S3.
- The most practical way to recognize the S3 or S4 is by listening with the bell of the stethoscope, which is useful to appreciate these lower frequency sounds, and then to listen with the diaphragm of the stethoscope, which cuts off the lower frequency sounds. Thus the S3 or S4 becomes muffled or cannot be appreciated.
- This description applies to a left ventricular gallop. A right ventricular S3 gallop is best heard over the lower left sternal border or rarely below the xiphoid process. It is best heard with the bell and may be heard as the patient inspires. It is heard in patients with right ventricular systolic or diastolic failure and indicates elevated right ventricular diastolic pressure.

The Fourth Heart Sound (S4 or Atrial Gallop)

- This sound results from forceful atrial contraction against a ventricle with decreased compliance. "This change in compliance may be related to ventricular hypertrophy, ischemia, infarction, fibrosis, or increased afterload as in systemic or pulmonary hypertension."[3]
- It is a low-frequency sound occurring just before S1 and best heard with the bell. A left ventricular S4 is best heard at the apex with the patient lying on the left side and may be accompanied by a presystolic outward movement of the apex, which is palpable and visible. A right ventricular S4 may be heard at the left sternal border.

- It may also be heard in first degree A-V block. It is also commonly heard in *acute* mitral insufficiency following rupture of a chorda tendinea. "An Audible S4 is an unusual finding in the normal heart in patients under fifty years of age except in the presence of A-V block."[3]

Close attention is required to differentiate an S4 from a split S1. Proctor Harvey points out the following distinguishing features:

- A split S1 is heard at the left sternal border and not at the apex or base. In contrast to an S4, it is of higher frequency and is not affected by pressure with the bell of the stethoscope whereas an S4 becomes softer with increased pressure.[3]
- A right-sided S4 may be heard at the left sternal border and becomes more apparent with inspiration.
- A striking finding which, if present, may help dispel doubt about equivocal auscultatory findings is the presence of quadruple rhythm that is audible, palpable, and visible at the apex with the patient lying on the left side. This is the result of an S1, S2, S3, and S4 sequence. Focus should start with visually observing the overall rhythm rather than individual events and then focus on each separate sound and apical movement. This finding may be seen in dilated cardiomyopathy.
- When both an S3 and S4 are present and are close together, as when the heart rate is rapid, the combined sound closely simulates a diastolic rumble and has been mistaken for the murmur of mitral stenosis.

THE VENOUS PULSE AND VENOUS PRESSURE

Identification of the Venous Pulse

It is important to recognize the jugular venous pulses adequately and properly (take care in being certain that the pulse is venous in origin). To assess venous pressure it is necessary that the top of the venous column is appropriately identified. Correct evaluation of venous pulse and pressure often clarifies the diagnosis. The statement "There was no jugular venous distention (JVD)" is a summary but a more comprehensive description is optimal.

- The venous pressure should be determined by observing the internal jugular (IJ) pulse that appears as a diffuse pulsation of the overlying skin.
- The external jugular pulse may be a reliable indicator of venous pressure with attention to proper technique (see below).
- The pulsations may be more easily seen when their inward and outward movements are observed with the examiner's line of sight perpendicular to these pulsations.
- With the patient lying down with head elevation at a level to optimize the venous pulse, stand behind the head and slightly to the right side.
- The patient's chin should be turned slightly to the left when observing the right IJ.

- Though the right IJ is traditionally examined for a variety of reasons, the left IJ can be examined as well and may be useful in some patients.
- Shining a penlight tangentially across the neck may also enhance observation.

Distinguishing the Venous from the Carotid Pulse

- The venous pulse has a characteristic sharp inward movement whereas the carotid pulse has a sharp outward movement and is often the most useful differentiator of the two.
- The height of the venous column will usually vary depending upon degree of head elevation.
- It will often vary with different phases of respiration, normally falling slightly with inspiration.
- It may normally be seen to rise transiently during hand pressure on the periumbilical region.
- The venous pulse is often multi-phasic and rippling and *usually not palpable* whereas the carotid pulse is usually mono-phasic with a sharp palpable upstroke, sometimes with a shoulder.
- The venous pulse is often obliterated or markedly dampened by pressure with the thumb at the base of the pulsation.
- In severe tricuspid regurgitation, the pulsations may be vigorous and difficult to obliterate with pressure, and the top of the venous column may be difficult to identify. Inward and outward pulsations of the ear-lobes may be noted. These findings may closely simulate carotid pulsations. Observing the venous column with the patient sitting on the edge of the bed or even standing may be helpful in identifying the height of the column and distinguishing it from the carotid pulse in this setting.

Estimating the Venous Pressure

- Identify the top of the venous column as indicated by the top of the venous pulsations. The degree of elevation of the patient's head above horizontal is determined by the level at which the top of the column is best seen and not necessarily by an arbitrary angle such as 45 degrees.
- If the height of the venous column is equal to or lower than the sternal angle the venous pressure is normal.
- An elevation of the venous pressure is said to be present if the height of the venous column is two to three cm above the sternal angle.[3]

Elevation of jugular venous pressure (JVP) reflects an increase in right atrial pressure and occurs in heart failure, reduced compliance of the right ventricle, pericardial disease, hypervolemia, obstruction of the tricuspid orfice, and obstruction of the superior vena cava.[4]

Using the External Jugular (EJ) for Accurate Estimation of Central Venous Pressure (CVP)[6]

* JVP can be accurately estimated if the EJ contains venous pulsations.
* Starting at 30 degrees identify the EJ and occlude it at the base of the neck.
* Empty the vein in an inferior to superior direction.
* The height of the column that refills from below is the JVP in centimeters.
* If the EJ cannot be visualized or the column extends above your finger, adjust the bed height accordingly.

Venous Pulse Waves

* The "A" wave precedes the carotid pulse upstroke and first heart sound and is due to right atrial systole. It is followed by the "X" descent as the atrium relaxes and the right atrial floor descends.
* The "V" wave begins after the arterial pulse and is due to filling of the right atrium during systole. The subsequent "Y" descent follows the second heart sound and is related to the fall in right atrial pressure as blood flows through the tricuspid valve into the right ventricle.

Examples of Abnormalities of the Venous Pulse Waves

* Significant tricuspid regurgitation is characterized by the presence of a prominent "V" wave followed by a more rapid and prominent "Y" descent.
* A giant "A" wave may be seen in right ventricular hypertrophy, as in pulmonary hypertension.
* Intermittent cannon "A" waves may be seen in complete heart block when sinus rhythm is present or in ventricular tachycardia and may aid in the diagnosis of a wide complex tachyarrhythmia.
* The "A" wave is absent in atrial fibrillation.
* An increase or no fall in the venous pressure during inspiration is called the Kussmaul sign and is observed in patients with constrictive pericarditis, restrictive cardiomyopathy, right ventricular infarction, and also in patients with partial venacaval obstruction and pulmonary embolism.
* In constrictive pericarditis or restrictive cardiomyopathy, not only is the jugular venous pressure elevated but there is also a sharp "Y" descent.

MURMURS

Systolic Murmurs
See Table 1-3.

Innocent Murmurs

THE 4 S's
1. Short: Mid-peaking murmur that terminates before S2
2. Systolic: Any diastolic murmur should be considered abnormal until proven otherwise

3. **Soft:** Grade III or louder murmurs require further investigation
4. **S2 normal:** Normal splitting of the second heart sound suggests a physiologic murmur

Although these findings are characteristic, the diagnosis of innocent murmur is one of exclusion since a similar murmur may be heard in pathologic conditions such as atrial septal defect and aortic and pulmonary stenosis.

The characteristic fixed splitting of the second heart sound in atrial septal defect is not heard with innocent murmurs. If there is doubt about the presence of fixed splitting when splitting is narrowly split in expiration, listening with the patient standing may be helpful. When standing, narrow splitting of S2 in expiration may become single and this makes atrial septal defect unlikely.

TABLE 1-3	Pan-systolic murmurs		
	Mitral Regurgitation	**Tricuspid Regurgitation**	**Ventricular Septal Defect**
Location	Usually best heard at the apex and may radiate to the midaxillary line or subscapular area and less commonly to the base	Left lower sternal border or apex	Left lower sternal border
Respiratory variation	Minimal variation or louder on expiration	Increased with inspiration	No change with inspiration
Other features	S3 is often present if hemodynamically significant. Same intensity after a pause (premature atrial contraction [PAC], PVC, or aortic stenosis [AS]) which can help differentiate it from AS in which the intensity after a pause increases	S3 if right ventricular diastolic pressure is elevated (decompensated) Large V wave, rapid Y descent, (and ventricularization of the JVP)	Very loud murmur if VSD is small (larger gradient) Often associated with a thrill

Systolic Murmur Complicating Myocardial Infarction

Not infrequently, a new systolic murmur will be noted in a patient with a recent myocardial infarction. The murmur may be detected incidentally or may accompany the onset of hypotension or congestive heart failure.

The differential diagnosis includes the following:

* Mitral regurgitation secondary to left ventricular dilation or ischemic papillary muscle. In these conditions, mitral regurgitation is often mild and the murmur may be early or late systolic.
* Mitral regurgitation due to rupture of a papillary muscle head: May not be loud or accompanied by a thrill at the apex, and the murmur may be absent in patients who develop cardiogenic shock.
* Ventricular septal defect due to rupture of the interventricular septum. Often accompanied by a murmur and thrill along the left sternal border.

Both acute VSD and ruptured papillary muscle are frequently accompanied by hypotension and heart failure. The murmurs may become softer or disappear as arterial pressure falls.

These conditions are often difficult to differentiate at the bedside. The presence of a systolic murmur in the setting of an acute myocardial infarction (AMI), particularly if new, is an indication to obtain a transthoracic echocardiogram as an emergency. This is a very useful tool to differentiate these conditions. It should be emphasized that pulmonary artery catheterization is not required to confirm the diagnosis of these complications of acute myocardial infarction.

Other Systolic Murmurs
See Table 1-4.

Diastolic Murmurs
See Table 1-5.

CARDIAC TAMPONADE

* When a patient is found to have a pericardial effusion, the presence or absence of cardiac tamponade becomes an immediate crucial issue.
* The hemodynamic consequences of cardiac tamponade such as low cardiac out-put result from cardiac compression from increased intrapericardial pressure usually due to accumulation of intrapericardial fluid. There is pandiastolic restriction of ventricular filling, and in advanced conditions, ventricles can be filled only during atrial systole. With decreasing

TABLE 1-4 Other systolic murmurs

Murmur	HOCM	AS	PS	MVP
Location	Heard best at lower left sternal border (LLSB) or apex	Right second interspace, left sternal border (LSB) apex	Left second interspace, LSB	Heard best at the apex
Radiation	Usually *not* to carotids, may radiate to right sternal border, apex and even to axilla	Usually to carotids, often to apex with musical quality	Can radiate to neck	More to LLSB, less frequently to the axilla
Timing	Mid-systolic and when secondary mitral regurgitation is present a long late systolic murmur is superimposed	Mid-systolic, later peaking murmur associated with ↑ severity of AS	Mid-systolic	Late systolic (may be confused with a diastolic murmur)
S2	In severe outflow obstruction, paradoxical splitting may occur	The second heart sound may be quite soft, single, or paradoxically split	Wide splitting of the second heart sound due to delay in P2 and the intensity of P2 may be obtunded	Usually normally split
Maneuvers	Increases in intensity during phase 2 of Valsalva, during post ectopic beat, or standing. Decreased in intensity during supine position, during squatting, and during phase 4 of Valsalva	Decreases in intensity with Valsalva or standing	Increases in intensity and duration during inspiration	The mid-systolic clicks and the onset of the late systolic murmur is closer to S1 on standing and during phase 2 Valsalva as ventricular volumes are decreased. Click and murmur moves → S2 (shorter) during squatting, supine position[3]

| Other notes | In contrast to valvular aortic stenosis, the carotid upstroke is brisk. Occasionally a bisferiens quality is appreciated.

A characteristic finding, if present, is a triple apical beat *(triple ripple)* as a result of a presystolic impulse, normal apical thrust, and mid-systolic outward movement of the apex[3] | With moderate to severe aortic stenosis, the carotid pulse may be slowly rising, may have an anacrotic character, and the amplitude may decrease. It should be appreciated that in elderly patients, even with severe calcific aortic stenosis, the carotid pulse features may be absent

An S4 may be heard at the apex accompanied by a visible and audible presystolic impulse | A prominent right ventricular lift | Often introduced by single or multiple systolic clicks as the prolapsed valve leaflets and chordal apparatus tenses[3]

The longer the murmur, the more severe the regurgitation |
|---|---|---|---|---|

HOCM, hypertrophic obstructive cardiomyopathy; AS, aortic stenosis; PS, pulmonary stenosis; MVP, mitral valve prolapse; RSB, right sternal border; LSB, left sternal border; LLSB, lower left sternal border

TABLE 1-5 Diastolic murmurs

Murmur	MS	AR	PR	Dock Murmur[7]
Location	Apex or just medial to the apex, best heard with bell in left lateral decubitus position (may be very localized)	RSB or LSB apex. Best heard with diaphragm in seating and leaning forward position, during held expiration	LSB with diaphragm	LSB, localized often to second or third interspace
Quality	Low pitch, rumbling	High pitched	High pitched	High pitched
Timing	Mid-diastolic with pre-systolic accentuation	Early diastolic decrescendo	Early diastolic decrescendo	Early diastolic
Maneuvers	S2→OS interval widens with standing or Valsalva,[2] shortens with tachycardia, in presence of mitral regurgitation, aortic stenosis, and regurgitation. Murmur increases in intensity and relative duration with exercise, during pregnancy, and with volume overload	Increases in intensity with exercise or isometric hand grip	Increases in intensity during inspiration	Increases in intensity with hand grip

Other	Loud S1 in early MS, may diminish in advanced disease if the mitral valves are heavily calcified and immobile	Diastolic murmur identical to MS may be heard at the apex (Austin Flint murmur). Presystolic component is usually absent (vs. MS),with vasodilator such as amyl nitrite decreasing intensity and duration of the Austin Flint murmur	Can increase in intensity with inspiration	This murmur is described in LAD stenosis and represents turbulent flow through the vessel in diastole
	OS vs. split S2: More likely OS if louder at apex than base			Very rare, need to exclude valvular lesions to make the diagnosis
	S2→OS interval shortens with increasing severity			
	Associated loud P2, RV heave of pulmonary hypertension and secondary tricuspid regurgitation signify significant disease	Soft S1 secondary to premature closure of the mitral valve indicates severe AR		

Diastolic Flow Murmurs: A diastolic rumbling murmur similar to that heard in stenosis of the tricuspid or mitral valve may be heard because of increased flow in the absence of obstruction. Examples include atrial septal defect and mitral regurgitation. Similarly, a third heart sound or summation gallop (S3, S4) may simulate a diastolic rumble suggesting a stenotic valve.

MS, mitral stenosis; AR, aortic regurgitation; PR, pulmonary regurgitation; RSB, right sternal border; LSB, left sternal border

- stroke volume, hypotension and reflex tachycardia result. With increasing intrapericardial pressure, right atrial pressure increases to maintain cardiac filling. This compensatory increase in right atrial pressure may become inadequate when intrapericardial pressure increases more than 20 mm Hg. Thus shock syndrome occurs when right atrial pressure approaches 20 mm Hg.
- It has been thought that the gold standard for cardiac tamponade is the invasive demonstration of elevated and equal intra-pericardial, right atrial, pulmonary artery diastolic, and pulmonary capillary wedge pressures at the time of pericardiocentesis coupled with a significant increase in cardiac output post-pericardiocentesis.[9] However, in clinical practice it is not necessary.
- Echocardiography is the non-invasive procedure of choice for the detection of *pericardial effusion*;[9] it is highly sensitive and specific for the diagnosis of tamponade.
- Several echocardiographic findings including systolic right atrial collapse, diastolic right ventricular collapse, inferior vena caval plethora, and respirophasic exaggeration of flow velocities across the mitral and tricuspid valves are highly suggestive of cardiac tamponade when the pre-test probability of tamponade is high.[8]
- In patients with cardiac tamponade, elevated jugular venous pressure, tachycardia, and pulsus paradoxus are almost invariably present. Rarely pulsus paradoxus may not be present with patients in shock; however, in these patient's there is almost always right ventricular collapse by echocardiography.[9] Auscultatory alternans and electrical alternans are occasionally present. It needs to be appreciated that the patient may have dyspnea; hemodynamic pulmonary edema is characteristically absent (see Table 1-6).

TABLE 1-6	Cardiac tamponade[9]		
History	Sensitivity (%)	Physical Finding	Sensitivity (%)
Dyspnea	88	Pulsus paradoxus >10 mm Hg	82
Chest pain	20	Tachycardia	77
Fever	25	Elevated JVP	76
		Diminished Heart Sounds	28
		Hypotension (SBP <120 mm Hg)	30

TABLE 1-7 Operating characteristics of the arterial line pulsus in patients with known effusion[9]

	Sensitivity (%)	Specificity (%)	LR + (95% CI)	LR − (95% CI)
Pulsus >10	98	70	3.3 (1.8–6.3)	0.03 (0.01–0.24)
Pulsus >12	98	83	5.9 (2.4–14)	0.03 (0–0.21)

- Tamponade remains a clinical diagnosis and the mere presence of an effusion with some findings suggesting "hemodynamic compromise," while certainly meriting close evaluation, is not synonymous with the diagnosis of tamponade.

In a single study in which patients with a documented pericardial effusion were referred for pericardiocentesis and had intra-pericardial pressures and cardiac output changes measured, arterial line pulsus paradoxus were predictive of tamponade. Sensitivity and specificity of pulsus paradoxus are shown in Table 1-7[9]:

- These sensitivities and specificities predicted tamponade as defined by a >20% increase in cardiac output post-pericardiocentesis.
- A pulsus of >25 mm Hg was highly predictive of a >50% increase in cardiac output after pericardiocentesis.
- These patients were known to have a pericardial effusion; thus the stated sensitivity and specificity may not be applicable to patients who have not yet had an echocardiogram.
- Other conditions resulting in pulsus paradoxus include COPD, congestive heart failure, mitral stenosis, massive pulmonary embolism, severe hypovolemic shock, obesity, and tense ascites.[8]

REFERENCES

1. Topol EJ, et al. Textbook of Cardiovascular Medicine. Lippincott, Williams, & Wilkins. 2006.
2. Constant J. Bedside Cardiology. 5th ed. Philadelphia: Lippincott, Williams, & Wilkins: 1999: 147–148.
3. Chizner MA. Classic Teachings in Clinical Cardiology: A Tribute to W Proctor Harvey M.D. Cedar Grove, New Jersey: Lannec Publishing, Inc; 1996:125–126:137–139:140–1123.
4. Braunwald E. Heart Disease: A Textbook of Cardiovascular Medicine. 5th ed. Philadelphia: WB Saunders, 1997:19.

5. Forrester JS, Diamond G, McHugh TJ, et al. Filling pressures in the right and left sides of the heart in acute myocardial infarction. A reappraisal of central-venous-pressure monitoring. *AM J Med.* 1971;285(4):190–193.
6. Vinayak AG, Levitt J, Gehlbach B, et al. Usefulness of the external jugular vein examination in detecting abnormal central venous pressure in critically ill patients. *Arch Intern Med.* 2006;166(19):2132–2137.
7. Dock W, Zoneraich S. A diastolic murmur arising in a stenosed coronary artery. *AM J Med.* 1967;42(4):617–619.
8. Curtiss EI, Reddy PS, Uretsky BF, et al. Pulsus paradoxus: definition and relation to the severity of cardiac tamponade. *AM Heart J.* 1988;115(2):391–398.
9. Roy CL, Minor MA, Brookhart MA, et al. Does this patient with a pericardial effusion have cardiac tamponade? *JAMA.* 2007;297(16):1810–1818.

CHAPTER 2

Stress Testing

IAN BROWN AND DONALD SCHREIBER

BACKGROUND AND APPROACH

Stress testing is one diagnostic instrument currently available to medical professionals for the evaluation and risk stratification of patients with known or suspected coronary artery disease (CAD). Stress testing may be done with concurrent electrocardiogram (ECG) monitoring, nuclear scintigraphy, or echocardiography. Indeed, the different tests and the wide variety of patients tested have made stress testing an increasingly complex and challenging area for practitioners. This chapter is aimed at providing the reader with an enhanced understanding of the subject. The first portion of this chapter examines exercise stress testing, describing which patients would benefit from exercise stress tests, the appropriate timing for these tests, and test protocols. The next section details pharmacologic and imaging alternatives, reviewing the indications for each and comparing the different modalities. The final section gives guidelines on interpretation of stress test results.

INDICATIONS

Stress tests have two primary indications: to diagnose CAD and to risk-stratify patients with known CAD.

Diagnosis of Obstructive CAD

For patients with symptoms of chest pain, or possible anginal equivalent, the medical provider reviews the history, physical, and ECG to help establish the likelihood that symptoms are due to CAD (Table 2-1). If the diagnosis is unclear, the physician can use a stress test to assist in the diagnosis of CAD.[1]

Stress tests are most useful in patients with intermediate pretest probability of CAD. If the patient has a high pretest probability of CAD, then the results of a stress test are not likely to change the management. If the patient has a low pretest probability, then the frequency of false positive tests may lead to overtreatment and/or unnecessary procedures. Note that in Table 2-1,

TABLE 2-1		Pretest probability of CAD			
Age	Gender	Typical/ Definitive angina pectoris	Atypical/ Probable angina pectoris	Nonanginal chest pain	Asymptomatic
30–39	Male	Intermediate	Intermediate	Low	Very Low
	Female	Intermediate	Very Low	Very Low	Very Low
40–49	Male	High	Intermediate	Intermediate	Low
	Female	Intermediate	Low	Very Low	Very Low
50–59	Male	High	Intermediate	Intermediate	Low
	Female	Intermediate	Intermediate	Low	Very Low
60–69	Male	High	Intermediate	Intermediate	Low
	Female	High	Intermediate	Intermediate	Low

From Gibbons RJ, Balady GJ, Timothy Bricker J, et al. ACC/AHA 2002 guideline update for exercise testing: A report of the American College of Cardiology/American Heart Association Task Force on Practice Guidelines (Committee to Update the 1997 Exercise Testing Guidelines). 2002; and from Diamond G, Forrester J. Analysis of probability as an aid in the clinical diagnosis of coronary-artery disease. *N Engl J Med.* 1979;300:1350–1358.

a 40-year-old male with a clinical diagnosis of nonanginal chest pain is still considered intermediate pretest probability for CAD. This underscores the limitations of clinical evaluation for ruling out CAD. Table 2-2 lists indications for exercise stress testing.

Stress tests also play an important role in evaluating CAD in the context of preoperative risk evaluation. Stress testing is most useful in patients with intermediate clinical cardiac risk who either have poor functional capacity (<4 METS) or who have better functional capacity (≥4 METS) but are undergoing a high-risk surgical procedure. Stress testing is also useful in patients who are in a low clinical cardiac risk group but have poor functional capacity and are undergoing a high-risk surgical procedure. A stepwise approach to preoperative cardiac risk evaluation for non-cardiac surgery is explored elsewhere.[4]

Risk Assessment in Patients with Symptoms or History of CAD

In patients with suspected or confirmed CAD, stress tests may be used for risk assessment: to develop a prognosis, and to help guide treatment. Table 2-3 shows indications for stress tests in these patients.

TABLE 2-2	Indications for exercise testing to diagnose obstructive CAD

Class I (Evidence and/or General Agreement that Procedure is Useful)

* Patients with an intermediate pretest probability of CAD on basis of gender, age, and symptoms (Table 2-1)

Class IIa (Weight of Evidence/Opinion is in Favor of Usefulness)

* Patients with vasospastic angina

Class IIb (Usefulness Less Well Established)

* Patients with high pretest probability of CAD
* Patients with low pretest probability of CAD
* Patients with <1 mm of baseline ST depression taking digoxin
* Patients with ECG criteria for LVH with <1 mm of ST depression

Class III (Evidence/Opinion that Procedure is Not Useful and May be Harmful)

* Patients with any of the following baseline ECG abnormalities:
* Pre-excitation syndrome (e.g., WPW)
* Electronically paced ventricular rhythm
* >1 mm resting ST depression
* Complete LBBB

ECG, electrocardiogram; LVH, left ventricular hypertrophy; WPW, Wolff-Parkinson-White; LBBB, left bundle branch block. From Gibbons RJ, Balady GJ, Timothy Bricker J, et al. ACC/AHA 2002 guideline update for exercise testing: A report of the American College of Cardiology/American Heart Association Task Force on Practice Guidelines (Committee to Update the 1997 Exercise Testing Guidelines).

Long-Term Risk Assessment

Stress tests are useful to help predict survival. Risk stratification is improved when the stress test augments the history of the patient and the description of the pain. There are many risk stratification schemes based on electrocardiographic, hemodynamic, symptomatic and imaging parameters. These are reviewed in more detail in the last section of this chapter. High-risk patients may benefit from angiography, angioplasty, or revascularization.

Short-Term Risk Assessment

For patients presenting with symptoms of acute coronary syndrome (ACS)—that is, with unstable angina (UA) or myocardial infarct (MI)—stress tests are useful to predict short-term risk.

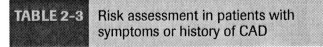

TABLE 2-3 Risk assessment in patients with symptoms or history of CAD

Class I (Evidence and/or General Agreement that Procedure is Useful)

- Patients undergoing initial evaluation with suspected or known CAD
- Patients with suspected or known CAD who present with significant change in status
- Low-risk UA patients, 8–12 hours after presentation, who have been free of active ischemic or heart failure symptoms
- Intermediate-risk UA patients, 2–3 days after presentation, who have been free of active ischemic or heart failure symptoms

Class IIa (Weight of Evidence/Opinion is in Favor of Usefulness)

- Intermediate-risk UA patients who have initial normal cardiac markers, repeat ECG without significant change, normal cardiac markers 6–12 hours after the onset of symptoms, and no other evidence of ischemia during observation

Class IIb (Usefulness Less Well Established)

- Patients with any of the following baseline ECG abnormalities:
- Pre-excitation syndrome (e.g., WPW)
- Electronically paced ventricular rhythm
- >1 mm resting ST depression
- Complete LBBB or any IVCD with QRS >120
- Patients with stable clinical course who undergo periodic monitoring to guide treatment

Class III (Evidence/Opinion that Procedure is Not Useful and May be Harmful)

- Patients with severe comorbidity likely to limit life expectancy and/or candidacy for revascularization
- High-risk UA patients

CAD, Coronary artery disease; UA, unstable angina; ECG, electrocardiogram; WPW, Wolff-Parkinson-White; LBBB, left bundle branch block; IVCD, interventricular conduction defect. From Gibbons RJ, Balady GJ, Timothy Bricker J, et al. ACC/AHA 2002 guideline update for exercise testing: A report of the American College of Cardiology/American Heart Association Task Force on Practice Guidelines (Committee to Update the 1997 Exercise Testing Guidelines). 2002.

The ability to rule out imminent ischemia is based on the test's negative predictive value. The negative predictive value of a stress test is dependent upon the specific test used; however, for low to moderate risk patients who rule out by enzymes and have an adequate negative exercise stress test, the short-term event rate is generally very low. Gibler et al. showed that only 1 of 1010 patients in a chest pain unit who ruled out for acute myocardial infarction and had a negative stress test died (cause unknown) within 30 days.[6] In another study, 0 of 374 patients had a combined endpoint of death or acute MI at 150 days.[7]

CONTRAINDICATIONS

Stress tests are generally safe procedures.[8] In a large national survey of exercise stress test facilities, encompassing both inpatient and outpatients, Stuard et al. enumerated complications including arrhythmias (<0.05%), infarcts (<0.04%), and death (<0.01%).[9] Looking at a higher risk group—632 hospitalized subjects evaluated for unstable angina symptoms—Stein et al. reported the combined incidence of MI and death within 24 hours of exercise testing as 0.5%.[10] Complications can be reduced by a careful history and physical, reviewing an ECG, and a pretest chest radiograph. Contraindications for exercise stress tests are shown in Table 2-4. Most of these contraindications are also applicable to pharmacologic stress tests.

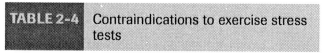

TABLE 2-4 Contraindications to exercise stress tests

Absolute

- Acute myocardial infarction (within 2 d)
- High-risk unstable angina
- Symptomatic or unstable arrhythmia
- Symptomatic severe aortic stenosis
- Uncontrolled symptomatic heart failure
- Acute pulmonary embolus or pulmonary infarction
- Acute myocarditis or pericarditis
- Acute aortic dissection

Relative

- Left main coronary stenosis
- Moderate stenotic valvular heart disease
- Electrolyte abnormalities
- Severe hypertension (>200 mm Hg/100 mm Hg)
- Tachyarrhythmias or bradyarrhythmias
- Hypertrophic cardiomyopathy or other outflow tract obstruction
- Mental or physical impairment leading to inability to exercise adequately
- High-degree atrioventricular block

From Gibbons RJ, Balady GJ, Timothy Bricker J, et al. ACC/AHA 2002 guideline update for exercise testing: A report of the American College of Cardiology/American Heart Association Task Force on Practice Guidelines (Committee to Update the 1997 Exercise Testing Guidelines). 2002.

TIMING OF STRESS TESTS

Stress tests should not be performed until the patient is clinically stable. Low-risk outpatients being evaluated for ACS symptoms should have a stress test within 72 hours.[1] The majority of low-risk patients admitted to the hospital can safely obtain their stress tests as outpatients. Current guidelines recommend that the stress test be obtained within 72 hours of discharge.[5] In general, outpatient stress tests for patients presenting via the emergency department (ED) with symptoms should be reserved for patients who are either at low risk for having ACS or low risk for short-term death or MI.[11,12] Outpatient stress tests are appropriate only for adherent patients.

Observation or chest pain units are increasingly common and provide a middle ground between inpatient and outpatient testing. Patient selection and management are based on accelerated rule-out protocols that ideally include stress testing.[5-7,10,13] These units have been shown to decrease unnecessary admissions, reduce the rate of missed MIs, reduce costs, and increase patient satisfaction.

STRESS TEST PROCEDURES: PRETEST PREPARATION

The patient should be informed of the purpose, risks, benefits, and details of the stress test procedure.[14] The patient should be instructed not to eat, drink, or smoke for 3 hours before the exam. Patients undergoing an exercise stress test should be instructed to wear comfortable clothing and footwear.

The physician should review the patient's medication list and decide what medications should be discontinued for the test. It is usually recommended that patients hold their dose(s) of beta-blocker 24–48 hours prior to exercise stress testing. A beta-blocker may blunt the chronotropic response to exercise and prevent the patient from reaching their target heart rates. This limits the diagnostic utility of the stress test. However, if there is risk involved in discontinuing beta-blocker therapy, there is some evidence to support that exercise tolerance or diagnostic accuracy is not affected.[15] In addition, the stress test can be used to test the medical management regimen that may include beta-blockers.

STRESS TEST ALTERNATIVES AND ENHANCEMENTS

Pharmacologic agents can be substituted for physical exercise to cause increased myocardial work and myocardial oxygen demand. The two major categories of imaging—echocardiography and myocardial perfusion imaging—can be used as an adjunct to either an exercise or pharmacologic stress test to delineate the extent, severity, and location of myocardial injury. Figure 2-1 gives an overview of the clinical context of stress testing, and provides a guide to the type of stress test that may be appropriate.

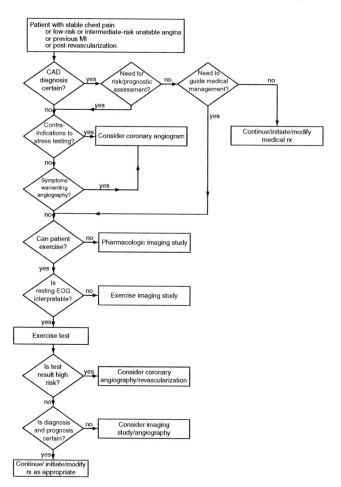

FIGURE 2-1 Clinical context for exercise testing for patients with coronary heart disease. ACC/AHA practice guidelines.[1] CAD, Coronary artery disease.

SPECIFIC THERAPIES

Exercise versus Pharmacology

For an exercise stress test, the patient must be able to use the available exercise equipment (usually a treadmill, or less often in the United States, a cycle ergometer) to elevate the heart rate to $\geq 85\%$ of predicted maximum heart rate ($HR_{Max} = 220 - $ age). If the patient is elderly, has significant comorbidity (e.g., chronic obstructive pulmonary disease [COPD], arthritis), or has other physical or mental limitation that would limit the ability to exercise, a pharmacologic stress test should be substituted. Pharmacologic stress tests generally use accompanying imaging.

The two choices for pharmacologic agents are vasodilators or dobutamine (the latter with or without atropine). Adenosine and dipyridamole are the current vasodilators of choice. Both agents are equally effective. They increase the heart rate, decrease the blood pressure, and increase myocardial oxygen demand, but may cause bronchospasm. Caution is warranted if there is a history of asthma or COPD. They may cause worsening angina. Both are contraindicated in high-degree A-V block and sick sinus syndrome. The short half-life of adenosine has a theoretical advantage if potential side effects are a concern. Theophylline and ideally caffeine must be withheld for 24 hours before the procedure. Calcium channel blockers, and nitroglycerin should ideally be withheld for 24 hours and beta-blockers for 48 hours, as they decrease the sensitivity of pharmacologic myocardial perfusion imaging.[18-20]

A dobutamine stress test is preferred in patients with history of bronchospasm or recent use of a methylxanthine. Dobutamine, an inotropic and chronotropic agent, is usually used in conjunction with echocardiography imaging but can also be used with myocardial perfusion imaging (MPI). Beta-blockers should be withheld for 24–48 hours.[21,22] unless the indication for the test is to evaluate the effectiveness of a medical regimen. Specific contraindications to a dobutamine stress test include the following:[18]

* Ventricular arrhythmias
* Recent MI (one to three days)
* ACS
* Hemodynamically significant left ventricular outflow tract obstruction
* Aortic aneurysm or aortic dissection
* Systemic hypertension.

The accuracy of a dobutamine stress echo is comparable to both adenosine and dipyridamole MPI (sensitivity $\sim$80%–90% and specificity $\sim$75%–85%). The choice of pharmacologic agent often has more to do with local expertise and individual patient characteristics rather than the advantages of each agent.[23] Since exercise tolerance and symptoms during exercise are important prognostic factors (see below), a submaximal exercise test can be combined with a pharmacologic protocol.[18,24-26]

Imaging

Moderate-risk patients, and any patients for whom there is a need to localize ischemia or assess the viability of myocardium, benefit from imaging in addition to ECG testing. For low-risk patients with normal ECGs who are not on digoxin, a standard (exercise) ECG stress test without imaging is sufficient.[1,27] However, there are guidelines[28] that recommend stress imaging in the risk stratification of low-risk as well as moderate-risk patients with symptoms. A stress test patient who has any of the following ECG abnormalities that can make ECG interpretation difficult (including low-risk patients) may benefit from an imaging modality:

* ST depression >1 mm
* Left bundle-branch block
* Intraventricular conduction delay with a QRS >120 ms
* Ventricular paced rhythm
* Pre-excitation syndrome

If imaging were not used, these pre-existing ECG abnormalities would limit the ECG diagnosis of ischemia.[1]

Myocardial perfusion imaging or echocardiography can be used with an exercise or a pharmacologic protocol depending on the patient's capability to exercise.

MPI can be done with positron emitting tomography (PET) scanning, single photon emission computed tomography (SPECT) imaging, or planar imaging. Stress PET imaging, while more sensitive, is considerably more expensive[23] and less readily available than SPECT imaging (Table 2-5). The only class I recommendation for an adenosine or dipyridamole perfusion PET is for cases where a SPECT scan produced equivocal results.[28] SPECT MPI, while still occasionally referred to as "thallium" MPI, is now usually done with a technetium isotope—sestamibi, tetrofosmin, or teboroxime—due to shorter half-life (lower radiation exposure and ability to use higher doses) with technetium, and to the high false-positive rates associated with thallium attenuation in soft tissue. SPECT imaging is considered to be superior to planar imaging.[23,29]

Echocardiograms are used to detect the presence of CAD and to risk-stratify patients. An echocardiogram can localize the area of ischemia by identifying segments with wall motion abnormalities such as hypokinesis or akinesis. If the echocardiogram is used in conjunction with an exercise stress test, the patient must move quickly from the point of peak exercise to an exam table where the echocardiogram can be performed and prior to the resolution of any ischemia that may be present. Echocardiograms are somewhat quicker to perform and less expensive than MPIs, but are more dependent on the sonographer's skills.

TABLE 2-5	Cost and accuracy of imaging modalities		
	1996 Cost	Sensitivity (%)	Specificity (%)
PET MPI	$1,500	91	82
SPECT MPI	$475	88	77
Adenosine		90	75
Dipyridamole		89	65
Dobutamine		82	75
Planar thallium MPI	$221	79	73
Stress echocardiography	$265	76	88
Adenosine		72	91
Dipyridamole		70	93
Dobutamine		80	84
Exercise electrocardiography	$100	68	77
Coronary artery bypass graft (CABG)	~$32,500		
MI: single admission	$7,415		
Catheterization with angiogram	$1,810		
Percutaneous coronary intervention (PCI)	$11,685		

Modified from Garber AM, Solomon NA. Cost-effectiveness of alternative test strategies for the diagnosis of coronary artery disease. *Ann Intern Med.* 1999;130:719–728; and Kim C, Kwok YS, Heagerty P, et al. Pharmacologic stress testing for coronary disease diagnosis: A meta-analysis. *Am Heart J.* 2001;142:934–944. These numbers reflect the average taken over all studies in the meta-analysis.

Patient variables can influence the choice of imaging modalities. In patients with left ventricular hypertrophy, stress echocardiograms have a superior specificity.[31] Vasodilator stress MPI is superior to exercise stress MPI or stress echo in patients with left bundle branch block or paced ventricular rhythms.[27] MPI is preferred if the patient's body habitus creates a poor echocardiographic acoustic window.

The choice of imaging modality is usually based on local expertise and availability rather than individual test characteristics. The sensitivity and specificity of these tests are given in Table 2-5. Some studies have shown that SPECT MPI has a higher sensitivity than echocardiography, while others have shown the two modalities to have comparable sensitivities. As expected, higher sensitivities are found in populations with higher prevalence and/or severity of disease. The specificity of stress echocardiography is slightly higher than for MPI.[23,31,32] These two options have similar performance characteristics for risk stratification and predicting outcomes.[33]

In addition to these two established imaging modalities, stress testing with magnetic resonance imaging (MRI) has shown encouraging results. It can be combined with either dobutamine or a vasodilator. In one study, sensitivity, when compared to dobutamine stress echo, was significantly higher, 86.2% versus 74.3%, and specificity was 85.7% versus 69.8%.[34] In addition to being accurate in diagnosing ischemic heart disease, MRI shows promise of having prognostic power.[35]

TEST INTERPRETATION

The provider must first determine whether the study was adequate. For the exercise portion of a stress test, the heart rate ideally should reach 85% or more of the patient's predicted maximum heart rate; lower heart rates increase the probability of a false negative result. For echocardiographic studies, satisfactory acoustic windows must be obtained to evaluate cardiac wall motion.

What is considered a positive or negative result on a stress test is somewhat arbitrary and depends on the desired sensitivity versus specificity of the test.[1] Predictors of adverse outcomes can be physiologic, electrocardiographic, or imaging abnormalities (Table 2-6).[36,37] Any one of these findings constitutes a poor prognosis. Not surprisingly, the inability to exercise is the strongest physiologic predictor of adverse cardiac outcomes. Downsloping ST segment depression, particularly in lead V5, is the strongest electrocardiographic predictor. Decreased left ventricular function is the strongest imaging predictor.[1]

The provider is not limited to considering these factors individually; there are tools available that allow prediction of mortality using multiple prognostic factors. Perhaps the best-established of these tools is the Duke Treadmill Score (DTS), which incorporates the depth of ST depression, the length of time on the treadmill, and the presence of angina (DTS = exercise time − [5 * ST deviation] − [4 * exercise angina]) to quantify a 5-year survival rate.[38-40] The DTS is a well-validated tool that is easy to use, but has some limits: it considers only three variables, and is somewhat dependent on patient morphology. It is most useful as a predictor when the score is either particularly high or low. These scores can be augmented with imaging information. Table 2-7 is an example of a risk stratification scheme that combines information from various aspects of the stress test, including echocardiographic imaging and the Duke treadmill score.[27]

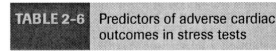

TABLE 2-6 Predictors of adverse cardiac outcomes in stress tests

Exercise

* Poor exercise capacity (<5 METs)
* Exercise-induced angina (particularly if test-limiting)
* Abnormally low peak systolic blood pressure (<130 mm Hg)
* Fall in the systolic blood pressure during exercise
* Chronotropic incompetence (<85 % of the age-predicted max HR)

Echocardiography

* Rest images
* New wall motion abnormality
* Stress images
* Stress-induced left ventricular abnormality
* Reversible dyssynergy
* Decreased wall thickening
* Decreased global left ventricular ejection fraction
* Increased LV end-systolic volume
* Reversible (or biphasic) segmental wall motion abnormality

Myocardial Perfusion

* Number and/or location of reversible defects
* Magnitude (severity and extent) of stress defects
* Lung uptake of isotope
* Transient ischemic left ventricle cavity dilation after exercise
* Delayed redistribution

EKG

* ≥ 1 mm horizontal or down sloping ST depression or elevation
* ≥ 2 mm of ischemic ST depression at a low workload (HR ≤ 130 bpm, or stage 2 or less)
* Early onset (stage 1) or prolonged duration (>5 min) of ST depression
* Multiple leads (>5) with ST depression
* ST segment elevation (in leads without pathologic Q waves and not in a VR)
* Ventricular couplets or tachycardia at a low workload or during recovery
* ST/HR slope (6 microV/beat per min)

Combined Exercise and EKG

* Elevated treadmill score (e.g., Duke)

Adapted from Weiner D. Exercise ECG testing to determine prognosis of coronary heart disease. In: *UpToDate*; 2006.

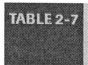 **TABLE 2-7** Prognosis based on Duke treadmill score and echocardiographic findings

High Risk (>3% Annual Mortality)

- Severe resting left ventricular dysfunction (LVEF <35%)
- High-risk treadmill score (score ≤−11)
- Severe exercise left ventricular dysfunction (exercise LVEF <35%)
- Echocardiographic wall motion abnormality (involving >2 segments) developing at low dose of dobutamine (≤10 mg/kg/min) or at a low heart rate (<120 bpm)
- Stress echocardiographic evidence of extensive ischemia

Intermediate Risk (1%–3% Annual Mortality)

- Mild/moderate resting left ventricular dysfunction (LVEF = 35%–49%)
- Intermediate-risk treadmill score (−11 < score <5)
- Limited stress echocardiographic ischemia with a wall motion abnormality only at higher doses of dobutamine involving ≤2 segments

Low Risk (<1% Annual Mortality)

- Low-risk treadmill score (score ≥5)
- Normal stress echocardiographic wall motion or no change of limited resting wall motion abnormalities during stress (unless high treadmill score)

LVEF, left ventricular ejection fraction adapted from Gibbons RJ, Chatterjee K, Daley J, et al. ACC/AHA/ACP-ASIM guidelines for the management of patients with chronic stable angina: A report of the American College of Cardiology/American Heart Association Task Force on Practice Guidelines (Committee on Management of Patients With Chronic Stable Angina). *J Am Coll Cardiol.* 1999;33:2092–2197.

REFERENCES

1. Gibbons RJ, Balady GJ, Timothy Bricker J, et al. ACC/AHA 2002 guideline update for exercise testing: A report of the American College of Cardiology/American Heart Association Task Force on Practice Guidelines (Committee to Update the 1997 Exercise Testing Guidelines). 2002.
2. Gibbons LW, Mitchell TL, Wei M, et al. Maximal exercise test as a predictor of risk for mortality from coronary heart disease in asymptomatic men. *Am J Cardiol.* 2000;86:53–58.
3. Diamond G, Forrester J. Analysis of probability as an aid in the clinical diagnosis of coronary-artery disease. *N Engl J Med.* 1979;300:1350–1358.

4. Eagle KA, Berger PB, Calkins H, et al. ACC/AHA guideline update for perioperative cardiovascular evaluation for noncardiac surgery—Executive Summary: A report of the American College of Cardiology/American Heart Association Task Force on Practice Guidelines (Committee to Update the 1996 Guidelines on Perioperative Cardiovascular Evaluation for Noncardiac Surgery). *Circulation.* 2002;105:1257–1267.

5. Braunwald E, Antman EM, Beasley JW, et al. ACC/AHA 2002 guideline update for the management of patients with unstable angina and non-ST-segment elevation myocardial infarction: A report of the American College of Cardiology/American Heart Association Task Force on Practice Guidelines (Committee on the Management of Patients With Unstable Angina). 2002.

6. Gibler W, Runyon J, Levy R, et al. A rapid diagnostic and treatment center for patients with chest pain in the emergency department. *Ann Emerg Med.* 1995;25:1–8.

7. Mikhail MG, Smith FA, Gray M, et al. Cost-effectiveness of mandatory stress testing in chest pain center patients. *Ann Emerg Med.* 1997;29:88–98.

8. Gordon NF, Kohl HW. Exercise testing and sudden cardiac death. *J Cardiopulm Rehabil.* 1993;13:381–386.

9. Stuart R Jr, Ellestad M. National survey of exercise stress testing facilities. *Chest.* 1980;77:94–97.

10. Stein RA, Chaitman BR, Balady GJ, et al. Safety and utility of exercise testing in emergency room chest pain centers: An advisory from the Committee on Exercise, Rehabilitation, and Prevention, Council on Clinical Cardiology, American Heart Association. *Circulation.* 2000;102:1463–1467.

11. Braunwald E, Antman EM, Beasley JW, et al. ACC/AHA guideline update for the management of patients with unstable angina and non-ST-segment elevation myocardial infarction—2002: Summary Article: A report of the American College of Cardiology/American Heart Association Task Force on Practice Guidelines (Committee on the Management of Patients With Unstable Angina). *Circulation.* 2002;106:1893–1900.

12. Meyer MC, Mooney RP, Sekera AK. A critical pathway for patients with acute chest pain and low risk for short-term adverse cardiac events: Role of outpatient stress testing. *Ann Emerg Med.* 2006;47:435. e1–435.e3.

13. Amsterdam EA, Kirk JD, Diercks DB, et al. Exercise testing in chest pain units: Rationale, implementation, and results. *Cardiol Clin.* 2005;23:503–16, vii.

14. Pina IL, Balady GJ, Hanson P, et al. Guidelines for clinical exercise testing laboratories. A statement for healthcare professionals from the

Committee on Exercise and Cardiac Rehabilitation, American Heart Association. *Circulation*. 1995;91:912–921.

15. Herbert WG, Dubach P, Lehmann KG, et al. Effect of beta-blockade on the interpretation of the exercise ECG: ST level versus delta ST/HR index. *Am Heart J*. 1991;122:993–1000.

16. Fletcher GF, Balady G, Froelicher VF, et al. Exercise standards. A statement for healthcare professionals from the American Heart Association. Writing Group. *Circulation*. 1995;91:580–615.

17. Gibbons RJ, Balady GJ, Timothy Bricker J, et al. ACC/AHA 2002 Guideline update for exercise testing: Summary Article: A Report of the American College of Cardiology/American Heart Association Task Force on Practice Guidelines (Committee to Update the 1997 Exercise Testing Guidelines). *Circulation*. 2002;106: 1883–1892.

18. Heller GV. Pharmacologic stress myocardial perfusion imaging in the diagnosis and prognosis of coronary heart disease. In: Up-To-Date, ed. 15.1 ed; 2007.

19. Taillefer R, Ahlberg AW, Masood Y, et al. Acute beta-blockade reduces the extent and severity of myocardial perfusion defects with dipyridamole Tc-99m sestamibi SPECT imaging. *J Am Coll Cardiol*. 2003;42:1475–1483.

20. Sharir T, Rabinowitz B, Livschitz S, et al. Underestimation of extent and severity of coronary artery disease by dipyridamole stress thallium-201 single-photon emission computed tomographic myocardial perfusion imaging in patients taking antianginal drugs. *J Am Coll Cardiol*. 1998;31:1540–1546.

21. Heller GV, Kapetanopoulos A. Pharmacologic stress myocardial perfusion imaging: Testing methodologies and safety. In: *UpToDate*. 15.3 ed; 2007.

22. Shehata AR, Gillam LD, Mascitelli VA, et al. Impact of acute propranolol administration on dobutamine-induced myocardial ischemia as evaluated by myocardial perfusion imaging and echocardiography. *Am J Cardiol*. 1997;80:268–272.

23. Garber AM, Solomon NA. Cost-effectiveness of alternative test strategies for the diagnosis of coronary artery disease. *Ann Intern Med*. 1999;130:719–728.

24. Casale PN, Guiney TE, Strauss, HW, et al. Simultaneous low level treadmill exercise and intravenous dipyridamole stress thallium imaging. *Am J Cardiol*. 1988;62:799–802.

25. Pennell DJ, Mavrogeni SI, Forbat SM, et al. Adenosine combined with dynamic exercise for myocardial perfusion imaging. *J Am Coll Cardiol*. 1995;25:1300–1309.

26. Thomas GS, Prill NV, Majmundar H, et al. Treadmill exercise during adenosine infusion is safe, results in fewer adverse reactions,

and improves myocardial perfusion image quality. *J Nucl Cardiol.* 2000;7:439–446.

27. Gibbons RJ, Chatterjee K, Daley J, et al. ACC/AHA/ACP-ASIM guidelines for the management of patients with chronic stable angina: A report of the American College of Cardiology/American Heart Association Task Force on Practice Guidelines (Committee on Management of Patients With Chronic Stable Angina). *J Am Coll Cardiol.* 1999;33:2092–2197.

28. Klocke FJ, Baird MG, Lorell BH, et al. ACC/AHA/ASNC guidelines for the clinical use of cardiac radionuclide imaging—Executive Summary: A report of the American College of Cardiology/American Heart Association Task Force on Practice Guidelines (ACC/AHA/ASNC Committee to Revise the 1995 Guidelines for the Clinical Use of Cardiac Radionuclide Imaging). *Circulation.* 2003;108:1404–1418.

29. Fintel DJ, Links JM, Brinker JA, et al. Improved diagnostic performance of exercise thallium-201 single photon emission computed tomography over planar imaging in the diagnosis of coronary artery disease: A receiver operating characteristic analysis. *J Am Coll Cardiol.* 1989;13:600–612.

30. Kim C, Kwok YS, Heagerty P, et al. Pharmacologic stress testing for coronary disease diagnosis: A meta-analysis. *Am Heart J.* 2001;142:934–944.

31. Marwick T, D'Hondt A, Baudhuin T, et al. Optimal use of dobutamine stress for the detection and evaluation of coronary artery disease: Combination with echocardiography or scintigraphy, or both? *J Am Coll Cardiol.* 1993;22:159–167.

32. Fleischmann KE, Hunink MG, Kuntz KM, et al. Exercise echocardiography or exercise SPECT imaging? A meta-analysis of diagnostic test performance. *JAMA.* 1998;280: 913–920.

33. Olmos LI, Dakik H, Gordon R, et al. Long-term prognostic value of exercise echocardiography compared with exercise 201Tl, ECG, and clinical variables in patients evaluated for coronary artery disease. *Circulation.* 1998;98:2679–2686.

34. Nagel E, Lehmkuhl HB, Bocksch W, et al. Noninvasive diagnosis of ischemia-induced wall motion abnormalities with the use of high-dose dobutamine stress MRI: Comparison with dobutamine stress echocardiography. *Circulation.* 1999;99:763–770.

35. Jahnke C, Nagel E, Gebker R, et al. Prognostic value of cardiac magnetic resonance stress tests: Adenosine stress perfusion and dobutamine stress wall motion imaging. *Circulation.* 2007;115:1769–1776.

36. Weiner D. Exercise ECG testing to determine prognosis of coronary heart disease. In: *UpToDate;* 2006.

37. Yao S-S, Rozanski A. Principal uses of myocardial perfusion scintigraphy in the management of patients with known or suspected coronary artery disease. *Prog Cardiovasc Dis.* 2001;43:281–302.

38. Mark D, Shaw L, Harrell F, et al. Prognostic value of a treadmill exercise score in outpatients with suspected coronary artery disease. *N Engl J Med.* 1991;325:849–853.
39. Kwok JMF, Miller TD, Christian TF, et al. Prognostic value of a treadmill exercise score in symptomatic patients with nonspecific ST-T abnormalities on resting ECG. *JAMA.* 1999;282:1047–1053.
40. Mark DB, Hlatky MA, Harrell FE, et al. Exercise treadmill score for predicting prognosis in coronary artery disease. *Ann Intern Med.* 1987;106:793.

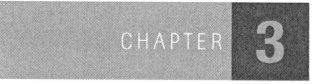

CHAPTER 3

Chest Pain and the Acute Coronary Syndromes

DAVID V. DANIELS, TODD J. BRINTON, AND DAVID P. LEE

BACKGROUND AND APPROACH

There are over 5 million emergency department visits each year in the United States for acute chest pain.[1] Annually, over 800,000 people experience an acute myocardial infarction (AMI), of which 213,000 die and half do so before reaching the hospital. In-hospital mortality in the pre-CCU era reached >30%. With the advent of the coronary care unit (CCU), mortality dropped to 15%, and in the modern era of percutaneous coronary intervention (PCI) with stenting, combination antithrombotic therapy, and routine use of adjunctive medical treatment, in-hospital mortality of ST segment elevation MI (STEMI) has reached a low of 6%–7%. In this chapter we review the initial recognition, triage, acute management, and definitive therapy across the spectrum of the acute coronary syndromes (ACS).

CLINICAL PRESENTATIONS

Acute Coronary Syndrome

The spectrum of acute ischemia-related syndromes ranges from unstable angina to acute myocardial infarction (MI), with or without ST elevation (see Figure 3-1), that are *secondary to acute plaque rupture or plaque erosion*. The clinical diagnosis relies on the combination of at least two of the following:

- History (angina or anginal equivalent)
- Acute ischemic electrocardiogram (ECG) changes
- Typical rise and fall of cardiac markers
- Absence of another identifiable etiology

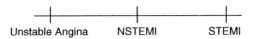

FIGURE 3-1 Spectrum of ACS.

Unstable Angina

Angina pectoris or ischemic symptoms with at least one of the following:

* Occurring at rest or with minimal exertion and usually lasting >20 minutes (if not interrupted by nitroglycerin)
* Severe pain of new onset (i.e., <1 month)
* Occurring with a crescendo pattern (i.e., more severe, prolonged, or frequent than previously)
* No evidence of myocardial infarction by biomarkers

Myocardial Infarction[2]

The typical rise and fall of troponin or creatinine kinase MB fraction (CK-MB) with at least one of the following:

* Ischemic symptoms
* Development of pathologic Q waves on the ECG
* ST elevation, depression or evolutionary EKG changes consistent with ischemia
* Post PCI (CK-MB 3× upper limit of normal)

Non-ST Segment Elevation MI (NSTEMI)

Criteria for MI in the absence of or with only transient ST elevation

ST Segment Elevation MI (STEMI)

Criteria for MI in the presence of persistent ST elevation indicative of myocardial injury

NQWMI/QWMI

The older literature makes reference to Q wave MI (QWMI) and Non-Q wave MI (NQWMI). The implication was that Q wave MI was associated with transmural infarction and Non-Q wave MI was limited to the subendocardium. Pathology studies have shown that Q waves are neither sensitive nor specific for transmural infarction. While there may be prognostic value in the identification of Q waves in patients with myocardial infarction, the modern terms STEMI and NSTEMI are preferred as they have more immediate implications with regard to acute management strategies (i.e., STEMI is triaged toward emergent reperfusion)

Causes of ST Elevation Other than AMI

Normal Variants

* Normal male pattern: Often with 1–3 mm of concave sinus tachycardia (ST) elevation greatest lead V2
* Early repolarization: Often with 1–3 mm of concave ST elevation, often with notching at the J point in V4
* Variant ST elevation with T wave inversion: Seen often in young black men, convex ST elevation, T wave inversion, thought to represent persistent juvenile T wave inversion + early repol, may look like STEMI

Other Pathology

* Left bundle branch block (LBBB): Typical pattern of LBBB present with anterior ST elevation
* Pericarditis: Diffuse ST elevation and PR depression, PR elevation in AVR, the ratio of ST elevation: T wave height (> 0.25 measured using PR segment as the baseline in this case) in V6 is highly sensitive and specific for the diagnosis of pericarditis
* Left ventricular hypertrophy with strain
* Hyperkalemia: Downsloping ST elevation associated with wide QRS, peaked T waves
* Pulmonary embolism: Sinus tachycardia, often anterior T wave inversions
* Takotsubo cardiomyopathy (apical ballooning syndrome)
* Brugada syndrome: Right bundle, downsloping ST elevation >2 mm isolated to V1 and V2

DIFFERENTIAL DIAGNOSIS OF CHEST DISCOMFORT

See Tables 3-1, 3-2, 3-3.

TABLE 3-1	Immediately life-threatening causes (must consider these every time)	
Disorder	History	Classic Findings
ACS	Substernal pressure with radiation to jaw, shoulder, arm, nausea, diaphoresis, often similar in character to previous angina. History of CAD, HTN, DM, hyperlipidemia, smoker, advanced age	-- Tachycardia, S4, new MR murmur or normal exam

(continued)

TABLE 3-1	*(Continued)*	
Disorder	**History**	**Classic Findings**
Aortic dissection	Acute onset, tearing CP, radiation to back, may be associated with stroke symptoms. History of HTN, Marfan syndrome	-- Classic clinical ACS with normal ECG -- May see ST elevation, classically inferior from RCA dissection -- Widened mediastinum -- Good *positive* predictors of the diagnosis: Pulse deficits and focal neuro findings with CP[3] -- New AI murmur -- Poor *negative* clinical predictors—if you think about it, exclude it
Pulmonary embolism	Acute onset, sharp, pleuritic CP, dyspnea, tachypnea. History/family history of DVT/PE/thrombophilia, malignancy, pelvic surgery, trauma, prolonged bed rest, travel, smoking, OCP	-- Always consider with hypoxia and a nl chest x-ray -- ECG most commonly sinus tach, also anterior TWI, new RBBB, RAD -- S1Q3T3 uncommon
Pneumothorax	Unilateral, sharp CP, pleuritic. History of trauma, asthma, COPD, mechanical ventilation, tall and skinny	-- Tracheal shift -- Lucency of chest x-ray -- Shock if under tension

TABLE 3-2	Urgent causes	
Disorder	**History**	**Classic Findings**
Pericarditis	Sharp, localized, relief with sitting forward	-- Friction rub -- Diffuse PR depression and/or ST elevation -- PR elevation in AVR -- ST elevation: T wave amplitude ratio in V6$\geq$ 0.25 very high sensitivity/specificity for acute pericarditis (baseline is end of the PR segment)[4]
Pulmonary HTN	DOE, anginal-like pain (? RV ischemia), history-middle age women>men	-- Elevated JVP, loud P2, parasternal lift, S4 -- Stigmata of R sided HF

Disorder	History	Classic Findings
		-- CXR with increased PA markings -- See chapter on PH
Myocarditis	CP, fever, malaise, viral prodrome	-- Can elevate troponins and focal myocarditis can even cause WMAs
Esophageal rupture	Pleuritic CP, History of violent vomiting, esophagitis	-- Chest x-ray with mediastinal air -- Hamman crunch on exam
Biliary tract disease	RUQ pain, postprandial, fever, history of gallstones, n/v	-- Murphy sign -- Jaundice if common duct -- Abnormal LFTs
Pancreatitis	Epigastric, radiates to back, alcoholic, History of pancreatitis or gallstones	-- LFTs in gallstone pancreatitis, Lipase
Pneumonia	Pleuritic, fever, cough, sputum production	-- Elevated WBC, fever -- Rhonchi, rales -- Chest x-ray with infiltrate

TABLE 3-3 Other causes

Disease	History	Classic findings
GERD	Long rest episodes with neg cardiac markers, burning, worse with recumbency, chocolate, caffeine, alleviated by antacids	-- Esophagitis on EGD -- Promptly relieved with GI cocktail (be careful here)
PUD/Gastritis	Epigastric burning, worse after meals, caffeine, stress	-- Epigastric tenderness -- Guaiac positive stools
Esophageal spasm	Substernal pain, aggravated with cold liquids	-- Often relieved with NTG (remember it's smooth muscle too!)
Costochondritis or chest wall trauma	Localized pain, history of trauma or recent viral illness	-- Tender to palpation
Herpes Zoster	Unilateral local pain, immunosuppression, HIV	-- Pain often precedes rash -- Make sure you look at the chest!

(continued)

TABLE 3-3 *(Continued)*		
Disease	History	Classic findings
Anxiety	History of panic attacks, GAD, Depression, PTSD, recent traumatic event, on antidepress-ants/benzodiazepines	-- This has to be a diagnosis of exclusion

ACS, acute coronary syndrome; CAD, coronary artery disease; HTN, hypertension; DM, diabetes mellitus; MR, mitral regurgitation; CP, chest pain; RCA, right coronary artery; DVT, deep venous thrombosis; PE, pulmonary embolism; OCP, oral contraceptive pill; CXR, chest x-ray; TWI, t wave inversion; RBBB, right bundle branch block; RAD, right axis deviation; COPD, chronic obstructive pulmonary disease; AVR, aortic value replacement; JVP, jugular venous pressure; P2, pulmonic second sound; DOE, dyspnea on exertion; RV, right ventricle; PA, pulmonary artery; RUQ, right upper quadrant; LFT, liver function test; WBC, white blood count; GERD, gastroesophageal reflux disease; EGD, esophagogastroduodenoscopy; PUD, peptic ulcer disease; NTG, hitroglycerin; GAD, general anxiety disorder; PTSD, post-traumatic stress disorder.

Other Disorders Presenting with Chest Discomfort and ECG Changes (+/− Biomarker)

* Takotsubo cardiomyopathy (apical ballooning syndrome)
* Coronary vasospasm (Prinzmetal angina)
* Coronary dissection

HISTORY

The history should be methodically taken and may be aided by remembering the "SOCRATES" mnemonic.

* Severity: The 1-10 scale is useful, functional limitations should be sought
* Onset: Be specific, can affect decisions about thrombolysis and PCI
* Character: Pressure versus sharp, pleuritic, tearing (aortic dissection)
* Radiation: Shoulder, jaw, arm, back
* Associated symptoms: shortness of breath (SOB), nausea/vomiting (N/V), palpitations, syncope
* Tempering factors: Rest, particular position (pericarditis—relief sitting forward)
* Exacerbating factors: Exertion, emotional state versus particular position
* Self assessment: Knowing the patient's fears is important for many reasons
* Also look for history of CAD, details of prior angiography, CABG or percutaneous coronary intervention (PCI), recent stress tests or echoes, other risk factors (DM, smoking, HTN, hyperlipidemia, cocaine use)

PHYSICAL EXAM

The physical exam in someone having an ACS may be entirely normal. Its purpose is to identify early complications of ACS as well as other possible etiologies of CP.

Look for:

* Hypotension/hypertension
* Arrhythmias
* Tachypnea or hypoxia
* Fever
* Bilateral SBP difference >15 mm Hg (think of aortic dissection)
* Asymmetric pulses and/or a focal neurologic exam (aortic dissection)
* Signs of heart failure (elevated JVP, S3, crackles, hemoptysis)
* New MR murmur (? papillary muscle ischemia)
* A new S4 in a patient with active CP is highly suggestive of ischemia
* Murmur of aortic stenosis, pulsus parvus et tardus
* Abdominal tenderness (biliary tract/pancreatic disease)
* Rectal exam—evaluate for melena or guaiac positive stool (? how aggressive to anticoagulate)
* Rash on the chest (Zoster), make sure to examine the chest on hospital day 2, the pain often precedes the skin findings!

LABORATORY EXAMS AND IMAGING

Cardiac Biomarkers
* Troponin I or T may be detectable as early as 2 hours after injury and CK-MB become detectable around 6 hours and are most sensitive at 10 hours
* Myoglobin may rise somewhat sooner but is nonspecific
* Must obtain serial tests q4-6 h for at least 10 hours after the start of CP to definitively r/o MI
* False positive in heart failure, significant hypertension, PE
* Look for typical rise and fall of enzymes in the context of CP and the ECG to make a diagnosis of NSTEMI
* Heart failure can be responsible for persistent low-grade elevation of troponin thought to be from elevated LVEDP leading to subendocardial necrosis often with normal CKs

Additional Labs
* WBC: Likely mildly elevated in AMI but may also establish infectious etiology for current state
* Hemoglobin: Anemia contributes to patients presenting with shortness of breath or angina
* Platelets: Severely depressed <50k levels may be a contraindication to PCI
* Electrolytes: Monitor for potassium and calcium abnormalities which may alter the ECG, Evaluate for infectious etiologies, electrolyte abnormalities

contributing to arrhythmias, biliary tract disease, or pancreatitis, if indicated

- Creatinine: Usually elevated in patients with longstanding HTN and DM. Elevated creatinine is a relative contraindication to angiography because of the risk of renal failure secondary to contrast nephropathy
- LFTs: Elevated in cases of hypotension due to shock or passive congestion due to elevated right-sided filling pressures. Also serum glutamic oxaloacetic transaminase/aspartate aminotransferase (SGOT/AST) can be elevated from an acute coronary syndrome as it is released from myocardial necrosis
- Urine toxicology: Should be obtained for all young or at-risk patients with concerning chest pain (cocaine-induced MI can result from thrombosis in addition to vasospasm and therefore reperfusion may be indicated)
- B-type natriuretic peptide (BNP): May be helpful in establishing the diagnosis of congestive heart failure (CHF) (see chapter on complications of AMI)

ECG
- Should be obtained within 5 minutes of arrival within the emergency department
- Make sure to label each ECG with the degree of pain
- Comparison to an old ECG can be helpful
- Repeat every 15 minutes ×2 if nondiagnostic, this has been shown to increase sensitivity
- Dynamic T wave and ST changes should greatly increase your suspicion for ACS
- Reoccurrence of CP should be re-evaluated with additional ECG recordings prior to giving NTG
- Obtain right-sided leads in those with inferior distribution injury to evaluate for RV injury or infarct
- Obtain posterior leads in patients with only anterior ST depression to r/o posterior wall STEMI

Chest X-ray
- Assess for a widened mediastinum and always consider aortic dissection
- Examine lung fields for evidence of a pneumonic process, pulmonary congestion, or pneumothorax
- Assess ribs and soft tissues for evidence of trauma
- Hypoxia/tachypnea with a clear CXR? Consider PE

Echo
- Useful test for evaluating systolic function, regional WMAs, effusion, valvular lesions, and to assess for complications of MI
- May be helpful in a high risk patient with ongoing CP and a nondiagnostic ECG or when the diagnosis of STEMI is in doubt

Helical CT of the Chest
* Used to assess for proximal PE and aortic dissection and to assess for other noncardiac etiologies of CP such as pneumonia or pulmonary mass
* Sensitivity and specificity are institutional and reader dependent
* Consider MRI if patient has CRI or is high risk for contrast nephropathy
* Different phase of contrast often needed for optimal evaluation of PE and aortic dissection

MANAGEMENT—NSTE ACS VERSUS STEMI

Differentiation of STEMI from non-ST-segment-elevation acute coronary syndrome (NSTE ACS) is critical to optimal management. These two entities have vastly different priorities as STEMI often involves a completely occluded artery and clinical data indicate that revascularization is both an emergency and that outcomes are tied to time to reperfusion. Management of NSTE ACS, both from a pathophysiologic and a clinical outcomes perspective focus on initial treatment with drugs that inhibit thrombosis and platelet aggregation usually in conjunction with a nonemergent early interventional approach and early adjunctive medical therapies. The major difference is the prioritization of treatments and the recognition of STEMI as a time-critical emergency.

TABLE 3-4	TIMI risk score (TRS) for UA/NSTEMI[11]	
Score calculation (1 point each)	Score	D/MI/Revasc @ 14 days
Age ≥65	0–1	5%
≥3 risk factors for CAD	2	8%
Known CAD (>50% stenoses)	3	13%
ASA use in past 7 d	4	20%
≥2 episodes of angina in 24 h	5	26%
ST deviation ≥0.5 mm	6–7	41%
(+) cardiac enzymes		
Add total points 0–7		

INITIAL EVALUATION AND RISK STRATIFICATION

See Figure 3-2 and Tables 3-4, 3-5 and 3-6.

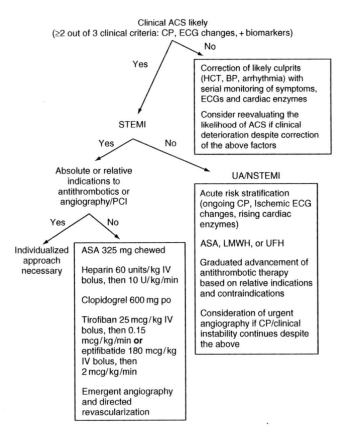

FIGURE 3-2 Approach to antithrombotic therapy in suspected ACS.

TABLE 3-5 UA/NSTEMI ACS risk stratification

	High risk (≥1 of:)	Low risk (all of:)
History	Prolonged anginal CP or CP relieved only with maximal medical treatment	New CCS II-IV angina in the past 2 weeks but NO CP >20 min
ECG	ST ↓ ≥0.5 mm in two contiguous leads or	No ST ↓ or TWI
	Deep TWIs >2 mm excluding AVR and V1	
Troponin	(+) Troponin	(−) Troponin
TIMI risk score	≥3	≤2

TABLE 3-6 Immediate NSTEMI ACS treatment strategies checklist

	Low risk	High risk
ASA 162-325 mg[5] (If allergy use Clopidogrel instead)	X	X
O_2 (To keep SaO_2 >90%)	X	X
B-Blockers[6] Lopressor 5 mg IVP q 5 min ×3 then 50 mg po q6h and titrate as tolerated. Harm likely in pts with significant CHF (see COMMITT CCS-2 below) *(Contraindicated HR <55, SBP <110 mm Hg, PR >0.24 S or advanced heart block, mod-severe CHF, severe asthma, cocaine ACS. If actively wheezing, consider Diltiazem for significant tachycardia)*	X	X
Nitroglycerin SL, Paste, IV *(Contraindicated in severe AS, HOCM, RV infarct, and Viagra/Levitra/Cialis use)*	X	X
Morphine Prn pain, anxiety	X	X
K >4.0 meq/dL, Mg >2.0 meq/dL Decreases risk of arrhythmias	X	X
DVT prophylaxis *(SQ heparin or LMWH prophylaxis for those not already on full anticoagulation)*	X	X

(continued)

TABLE 3-6	*(Continued)*		
		Low risk	High risk
Enoxaparin or UFH[7] Enoxaparin 1 Mg/Kg SC q 12 hr, UFH may be favored if urgent cath *(If Cr > 2.5, CrCl < 30 ml/min, or weight > 150 kg use UFH, relative contraindication: significant anemia, low plts)*			X
Clopidogrel[8] 600 mg po load then 75 mg daily *(Contraindicated with thrombocytopenia and caution with guaiac positive patients, caution if high likelihood of CABG, consult fellow/attending)*			X
GPIIB/IIIA inhibitor[9] *(Start immediately for STEMI. In NSTEMI benefit probably only in troponin + patients, PCI, and greatest benefit in diabetics, consult fellow/attending for guidance)*			X
High dose statin[10] Lipitor 40–80 mg po daily or Simvastatin 40–80 mg po qhs *(check baseline LFTs, lipid panel in am on all ACS patients)*			X
ACE inhibitor before discharge for ↓ EF or HF Captopril 6.25 mg po tid and titrate to goal 50 mg tid Ramipril 2.5 mg po and titrate to goal 5 mg po bid *(Especially with anterior MI or ↓ EF, contraindicated if hypotensive, ARF or ↑ K^+)*			X
Early coronary angiography and reperfusion (See chapter on angiography and PCI)			X

Adapted from the ACC/AHA 2002/2004 practice guidelines. (TIMI), thrombolysis in myocardial infarction

STEMI MANAGEMENT

As mentioned above, STEMI is often associated with a completely occluded coronary artery (>90%) and outcomes are directly tied to timeliness and adequacy of revascularization. The goal of reperfusion using PCI is a door-to-balloon time of <90 minutes in an experienced center and is preferred over thrombolysis when possible. If thrombolysis is employed the goal is a door-to-needle time of <30 minutes in the absence of contraindications (see below). Additional antithrombotic, antiplatelet, and adjunctive medical therapies are indicated in STEMI as above in NSTEMI ACS but should not delay reperfusion in any way.

PCI versus Thrombolysis in STEMI
See Table 3-7.

TABLE 3-7	PCI versus thrombolysis in STEMI

Angiography with directed PCI preferred	Thrombolysis preferred
Skilled PCI lab with surgical backup available (Door-to-balloon time <90 min) or rapid transport (<2 h) available to an experienced center	Early presentation (<3 h from onset of symptoms) with a delay (>2 h) to an invasive strategy
Cardiogenic shock	No appropriate PCI lab available
Contraindications to thrombolysis	No contraindications to thrombolysis
Late presentation: >3 h from pain onset	
Diagnosis of STEMI is in question	

Adapted from the ACC/AHA 2004 practice guidelines.

SPECIFIC THERAPIES

Thrombolytic Regimens
See Table 3-8.

Rescue PCI
Thrombolysis success is associated with resolution of chest pain, >50% resolution of ST elevations, hemodynamic stability, and reperfusion rhythms such as an accelerated idioventricular rhythm (do not treat unless unstable). Indications of thrombolysis failure include ongoing chest pain, hemodynamic instability <50% resolution of ST elevations, and malignant ventricular tachycardia. In such cases rescue PCI is the optimal management strategy, and if not locally available, arrangements for critical care air or ground transport to a tertiary center should be arranged.

Contraindications to Thrombolysis and Combination Antithrombotic Therapy
Antithrombotic therapy is associated with increases in the risk of major and minor bleeding and therefore decisions about appropriateness of therapy should also take into account relative contraindications so that a decision about the relative risks and benefits can be made. Remember that most patients with these contraindications were excluded from major clinical trials of advanced antithrombotic/antiplatelet therapy, and therefore bleeding rates in these trials likely underestimate bleeding in our population.

TABLE 3-8 Thrombolytic regimens

Drug	Dose	Notes	Adjunctive Therapy
Streptokinase	1.5 million units over 30–60 min	Inferior to TPA, patient may be refractory if prior exposure	ASA, +/− heparin
Alteplase – TPA	15 mg bolus IV push Then 0.75 mg/kg over 30 min (max 50 mg) Then 0.50 mg/kg over the next 60 min (max 35 mg)	Better outcomes compared to streptokinase (30 day mortality 6.3 vs. 7.3% in GUSTO-1)	ASA: 325 mg/d Heparin: 60 U/kg (max 4000 U), then 12 U/kg/h (max 1000 U/h) Clopidogrel: <75 years old 300 mg load then 75 mg/d >74 years old 75 mg/d
Tenecteplase – TNK	Single bolus IV push <60 kg = 30 mg 60–69 kg = 35 mg 70–79 kg = 40 mg 80–89 kg = 45 mg >90 kg = 50 mg	As effective as alteplase in ASSENT −2 with less noncerebral bleeding, single bolus easier to administer	
Reteplase	10 units over 2 min then repeat 10 unit bolus at 30 min	Similar outcomes to alteplase	

Also consider that patients with acute anemia, significant hyper- or hypotension, superimposed severe aortic stenosis, and other factors known to alter myocardial supply-demand relationships may not have plaque rupture as an etiology of myocardial infarction. Therefore, they may derive less benefit, and potentially more harm, from these therapies. The following are generally considered contraindications to thrombolytic therapy and should be considered individually for patients getting multiple antithrombotic and antiplatelet agents as well:

See Tables 3-9, 3-10, 3-11.

TABLE 3-9 Contraindications to thrombolytic therapy

Absolute	Relative
• Any prior intracranial hemorrhage	• History of chronic severe HTN
• Known cerebrovascular malformation (e.g., arteriovenous malformation [AVM])	• Severe HTN on presentation, systolic blood pressure (SBP) >180, DBP >110
• Known malignant intracranial neoplasm	• History of ischemic stroke >3 mo, other intracranial pathologies
• Prior ischemic stroke from >3 h to 3 mo	• Prolonged CPR >10 min
• Suspected aortic dissection	• Surgery <3 weeks prior
• Active bleeding diatheses (excluding menses)	• Recent <2–4 weeks of internal bleeding
• Significant closed head or facial trauma w/in 3 mo	• Noncompressible vascular punctures
	• Thrombocytopenia
	• Pregnancy
	• Active peptic ulcer
	• Current use of oral anticoagulation

Adapted from the ACC/AHA 2004 practice guidelines.

TABLE 3-10 TIMI Risk Score (TRS) for STEMI

Score Calculation	Points	Score	In-Hospital Mortality (%)
History of DM, HTN, or angina	1	0	0.8
Anterior STEMI or LBBB	1	1	1.6
Time to treatment >4 h	1	2	2.2
Weight <67 kg	1	3	4.4
HR >100	2	4	7.3
Killip class II-IV	2	5	12.4
Age ≥ 65–74	2	6	16.1
Age ≥ 75	3	7	23.4
SBP <100 mm Hg	3	8	26.8
		>8	35.9

TABLE 3-11 Post MI discharge checklist

Intervention	Comments
Cardiac rehabilitation	*Phase II as an outpatient with restrictions as indicated*
ASA 81–162 mg daily	*All patients without ASA allergy or contraindication*

(continued)

| TABLE 3-11 | *(Continued)* |

Intervention	Comments
Stress testing	*For patients who are not revascularized: Submaximal*
Plavix 75 mg daily	*At least 9–12 months after NSTEMI or STEMI w/o PCI. predischarge stress test or symptom limited ETT at 14-21* *Minimum 2 weeks s/p bare metal stent and 3 months s/p d post MI drug eluting stent Lifelong therapy probably if tolerated*
Post-discharge echo	*At 1 mo post d/c: Important especially in those with LV tolerated. dysfunction to assess for ICD criteria (EF <35%)*
Statin	*Target LDL <70 mg/dl w/LFTs and repeat lipid profile in 1 month*
Beta Blocker	*To target HR of 55–65 @ rest, consider Carveidolol if EF <40% post MI*
ACE –I or ARB	*Probably most useful with large anterior infarcts or those with post MI LV dysfunction (EF <40%). Target BP <130/80 for DM or CRI. Check BMP in 1–2 weeks[2]*
Nitroglycerin	*NTG SI for occasional angina. Isordil, Imdur, or nitro patch for patients with recurrent angina or medically treated obstructive CAD*
Aldosterone antagonist	*Indicated in post MI patients with an EF <40% and CHF. Must monitor K and renal function carefully or don't prescribe! at 1 week and 4 weeks*
Coumadin	*For patients with AF or documented LV thrombus. INR 2.0–3.0*
Diabetes management	*Target HbA1C <7.0%*
Smoking cessation	*All patients*
Cardiac Rehabilitation	*Phase II as an outpatient with restrictions as indicated*
Stress testing	*For patients who are not revascularized: Submaximal predischarge stress test or symptom limited ETT at 14-21 days post MI*
Post-discharge Echo	*At 1 month post d/c: Important especially in those with LV dysfunction to assess for ICD criteria (EF < 35%)*

Adapted from the ACC/AHA 2002/2004 practice guidelines.

LANDMARK CLINICAL TRIALS

See Tables 3-12 to 3-15.

TABLE 3-12 PCI and thrombolysis in STEM1

Intervention	Trial	Details
Streptokinase (S) vs. Placebo (P) Streptokinase + ASA (S+A) vs. Placebo (P)	GISSI-1 (Lancet, 1986[12]) ISIS -2 (Lancet, 1988[13])	Streptokinase → 18% RRR (P 13% S 10.7%) death 21 d, most benefit if tx w/in 1 h of symptoms **NNT = 44** Streptokinase + ASA → 42% RRR (P 13.2% S + A 8.0%) death @ 5 weeks **NNT = 20**
Primary PTCA (P) vs. Thrombolysis (T)	Metanalysis (JAMA, 1997[14]) n = 2606	PTCA → 34% RRR of (T 6.5% P 4.4%) death @ 30 d **NNT = 48**
Primary PCI w/stenting (P) vs. Thrombolysis (T)	Danami 2 (NEJM, 2003[15]) n = 1572	PCI w/stenting → 45% RRR (T 13.7% P 8.0) of death/MI/stroke @ 30 d compared with thrombolysis in patients transported from community hospitals w/in 2 h **NNT = 18**
Primary PCI w/Sirolimus drug eluting stent (D) + tirofiban vs. bare metal stenting (B) + abciximab	STRATEGY (JAMA, 2005[16]) n = 175	Sirolimus stent → 65% RRR (B 20% D 7%) TVR @ 8 mo **NNT = 8**

TABLE 3-13 PCI in NSTEM1

Intervention	Trial	Details
Early invasive (E) vs. selectively invasive (S)	Meta-analysis (JACC, 2006[17])	Early invasive → 25% RRR (S 6.5% E 4.9%) of death at 2 y **NNT = 63**
	Meta-analysis (JAMA, 2005[18]) n = 9212	Early invasive → 15% RRR (S 12.2% S 14.4%) D/MI @ 17 mo **NNT = 46**
	ICTUS (NEJM, 2005[19]) n = 1200	(Troponin positive subgroup) Early invasive → 30% RRR D/MI @ 17 mo **NNT = 25** No difference between early invasive and selectively invasive groups. n.b.: Both groups received background Enoxaparin and most got Clopidogrel and high dose statins up front. Crossover rate to diagnostic cath in the selectively invasive group was 53% during the index hospitalization and they remained in hospital for up to 12 days before stress testing.

TABLE 3-14	Antiplatelet and antithrombotics	
Intervention	**Trial**	**Details**
Aspirin vs. placebo	Canadian multicenter trial[ua/nstemi] (NEJM, 1985[5]) n = 555	ASA → 43% RRR all cause death @ 18 mo
	RISC[80% ua/nstemi] (Lancet, 1990[20]) n = 796	ASA → 64% RRR of D/MI @ 3 mo **NNT = 9**
	ISIS-2[56% STEMI] (Lancet, 1988[13]) n = 17,871	ASA → 23% RRR of death @ 5 weeks **NNT = 42** (Cost per life saved = $13!!)
Heparins (UFH or LMWH vs. placebo)	Metanalysis (Lancet, 2000[21]) n = 17,157	47% RRR of D/MI at 1 week (background: ASA) **NNT = 35**
Enoxaparin vs. UFH*	ESSENCE[ua/nstemi] (NEJM, 1997[7]) n = 3,171	Enox → 16% RRR of D/MI/Angina @ 14 d **NNT = 32** (30% revascularization rate, background ASA)
	INTERACT[ua/nstemi] (Circ, 2003[22]) n = 746	Enox → 56% RRR of D/MI @ 30 d in high risk ACS patients receiving eptifibatide **NNT = 25** (30% revascularization rate, background: asa, eptifibatide)
	SYNERGY[ua/nstemi] (JAMA, 2004[22]) n = 10,027	No difference between Enox vs. UFH at 30 d in patients managed with an early invasive approach. Small increase in major bleeding with Enox in those patients who crossed over from UFH→ Enox. (Background: ASA, Clopidogrel – 66%, 2b/3a – 57%)
Clopidogrel vs. placebo*	CURE[ua/nstemi] (NEJM, 2001[8]) n = 12,562	20% RRR of D/MI/Stroke @ 9 mo (80% medical management) **NNT = 48**
		Increase in major bleeding but NOT life threatening bleeds **NNH = 100**
	PCI-CURE (PCI treated subgroup of CURE)[ua/nstemi] (Lancet, 2001[23]) n = 2,658	Clopidogrel 300 mg loading dose and 75 mg/day vs. placebo → 34% RRR (P 4.4% C 2.9%) of D/MI @ 30 d in patients undergoing PCI for UA/NSTEMI (Average 6 d pretreatment prior to stent. Open label

Intervention	Trial	Details
		Clopidogrel was used from PCI to 30 d in 80% of patients, hence difference pretreatment) **NNT = 67**
	CREDO[ua/nstemi] (JAMA, 2002[24]) n = 2,116	Clopidogrel 300 mg loading dose prior to PCI vs. placebo strong trend ($p = 0.051$) of 39% RRR of D/MI/uTVR at 28 d if pretreated >6 h pre-pci. (All got open label Clopidogrel for 30 d poststenting, background: ASA, heparin, gp2b/3a 45%) *67% RRR if pretreated for >15 h* **NNT = 16**
Clopidogrel vs. placebo	PCI-Clarity (JAMA, 2005[25]) n = 1,863	Clopidogrel pretreatment vs. loading after angiography in 3 d postthrombolysis STEMI → 46% RRR (P 6.2% C 3.6%) of d/mi/stroke at 30 d (30% got GPIIB/IIIA inhibitor with PCI, additive benefit in this group rather than reduction in benefit) **NNT = 39**
GPIIB/IIIA vs. placebo *	ADMIRAL[stemi] (NEJM, 2001[26]) n = 300	Abciximab (A) → 60% RRR (P 14.6% A 6%) of D/MI/uTVR @ 30 d **NNT = 12**
	PURSUIT[ua/nstemi] (NEJM, 1998[9]) n = 11,000	Eptifibatide → 9% RRR of D/MI @ 30 d **NNT = 67**
	Metanalysis[ua/nstemi] (Lancet, 2002[27]) n = 31,400	2b/3a → 9% RRR (P 11.8% 2b/3a 10.8%) of D/MI @ 30 d **NNT = 100** (Benefit limited to + Trop or those that underwent revascularization within 30 days)
	Metanalysis of diabetics[ua/nstemi] (Circulation, 2001[28]) n = 6,458	2b/3a → 25 % RRR (P 6.2% 2b/3a 4.6%) of death in all pts @ 30 d **NNT = 63**
		2b/3a → 70% RRR of death in those undergoing PCI @ 30 d **NNT = 26**

* Studies showed benefit primarily in patients stratified as "High risk"
stemi Primarily STEMI patient population
nstemi Primarily NSTEMI patient population
RRR, relative risk reduction; NNT, number needed to treat; D/MI, death/MI

TABLE 3-15	Adjunctive medical therapy	
Intervention	**Trial**	**Details**
Acute beta blockade vs. placebo	Goteborg study *(Lancet, 1981[29])* n = 1,395	Metoprolol 15 mg IV, then total 100 mg po bid → 36% RRR (P 8.9% M 5.7%) of death @ 90 d **NNT = 32**
	ISIS-1 *(Lancet, 1986[30])* n = 16,027	Atenolol 5–10 mg IV then 100 mg po daily → 15% RRR of death @ 7 d **NNT = 143**
	TIMI 2B *(Circulation, 1991[31])* n = 1,434	Metoprolol 15 mg IV then total 100 mg po bid vs. metoprolol po starting day 6 → No difference in mortality or LV function, 50% RRR (P 5.1% M 2.7%) in re-infarction at 6 d
	COMMITT- CCS 2 *(Lancet, 2005[32])* n = 45,852	Metoprolol 15 mg IV then total 200 mg po a day → *No mortality benefit,* minimal reinfarction and VF benefit, increased risk of cardiogenic shock Reinfarction and VF NNT = 200 Cardiogenic shock overall NNH = 91 HR >110 NNH = 30 BP <110 NNH = 42 Killip III NNH = 18
Secondary prevention	CAPRICORN *(Lancet, 2001[33])* n = 1,959 Metanalysis *(NEJM, 1998)*	Pts with EF <40% post-MI, Carvedilol → 20% RRR (P 15% C 12%) mortality at 1.3 y **NNT = 34** βBs → 40% RRR of death @ 2 y **NNT = 11**
Statins secondary prevention	4S *(Lancet, 1994[34])* n = 4,444	In patients with CHD Simvastatin (S) → 30% RRR (P 12% S 8%) of death at 5 y **NNT = 25**
	TNT *(NEJM, 2005[35])* n = 10,001	Atorvastatin 80 mg vs. Atorvastatin 10 mg → 22% RRR (10 mg 10.9% 80 mg 8.7%) of death/MI/resuscitated cardiac arrest/stroke at 5 y. Avg ldl in 80 mg group = 77 mg/dL vs. 10 mg group = 101 mg/dL. AST/ALT elevations 1.2% in 80 mg group vs. 0.2% in 10 mg group.

Intervention	Trial	Details
Statins post ACS	PROVE IT – TIMI 22 Atorvastatin (A) 80 mg vs. pravastatin (P) 40 mg *(NEJM, 2004[36])* $n = 4,162$	Atorvastatin → RRR 15% (P 26% A 22%) of D/ACS/PCI/stroke @ 2 y **NNT = 26**
	MIRACL Atorvastatin (A) 80 mg vs. placebo *(JAMA, 2001[10])* $n = 3,086$	Atorvastatin → 16% RRR (P 17.4% A 14.8%) of death/mi/cardiac arrest/rehospitalization for ischemia at 16 weeks. Driven primarily by ischemia. **NNT = 39**
ACE inhibitor	SAVE – EF <40%[stemi] *(NEJM, 1992[37])*	Captopril (S) 50 mg TID vs. placebo → 19% RRR (P 25% C 20%) death @ 42 mo **NNT = 20**
ACE inhibitor	SAVE – EF <40%[stemi] *(NEJM, 1992[37])*	Captopril (S) 50 mg TID vs. placebo → 19% RRR (P 25% C 20%) death @ 42 mo **NNT = 20**
	SMILE – Anterior MI[stemi] *(NEJM, 1995[38])*	RRR 46% of Severe HF @ 6 weeks RRR 29% of death @ 1 y **NNT = 25**
	AIRE *(Lancet, 1993[39])* $n = 2,006$	Ramipril vs. placebo → 27% RRR (P 23% R 17%) of death at 15 mo **NNT = 17**
Aldosterone antagonist – Eplerenone	EPHESUS *(NEJM, 2003[40])*	Patients with EF <40% and clinical HF or DM, Eplerenone (E) 25 mg → 15% RRR (P 16.7% E 14.4%) of death @ 18 mo **NNT = 44**
K and Mg replacement	GISSI-2 *(Am J Card, 1998)*	OR 1.97 for VF if K<3.6

[stemi] Primarily STEMI patient population
[nstemi] Primarily NSTEMI patient population
RRR, relative risk reduction
OR, odds ratio
NNT, number needed to treat

REFERENCES

1. Fuster V, Alexander RW, O'Rourke RA. *Hurst's the Heart.* 11th ed. New York: McGraw-Hill Medical Publishing Division; 2004.
2. Alpert JS, Thygesen K, Antman E, et al. Myocardial infarction redefined—a consensus document of The Joint European Society of Cardiology/American College of Cardiology Committee for the Redefinition of Myocardial Infarction. *J Am Coll Cardiol.* 2000;36(3):959–969.

3. Klompas M. Does this patient have an acute thoracic aortic dissection? *JAMA.* 2002;287(17):2262–2272.
4. Ginzton LE, Laks MM. The differential diagnosis of acute pericarditis from the normal variant: New electrocardiographic criteria. *Circulation.* 1982;65(5):1004–1009.
5. Cairns JA, Gent M, Singer J, et al. Aspirin, sulfinpyrazone, or both in unstable angina. Results of a Canadian multicenter trial. *N Engl J Med.* 1985;313(22):1369–1375.
6. Freemantle N, Cleland J, Young P, et al. Beta blockade after myocardial infarction: Systematic review and meta regression analysis. *BMJ.* 1999;318(7200):1730–1737.
7. Cohen M, Demers C, Gurfinkel EP, et al. A comparison of low-molecular-weight heparin with unfractionated heparin for unstable coronary artery disease. Efficacy and Safety of Subcutaneous Enoxaparin in Non-Q-Wave Coronary Events Study Group. *N Engl J Med.* 1997;337(7):447–452.
8. Yusuf S, Zhao F, Mehta SR, et al. Effects of clopidogrel in addition to aspirin in patients with acute coronary syndromes without ST-segment elevation. *N Engl J Med.* 2001;345(7):494–502.
9. Inhibition of platelet glycoprotein IIb/IIIa with eptifibatide in patients with acute coronary syndromes. The PURSUIT Trial Investigators. Platelet glycoprotein IIb/IIIa in unstable angina: Receptor suppression using Integrilin therapy. *N Engl J Med.* 1998;339(7):436–443.
10. Schwartz GG, Olsson AG, Ezekowitz MD, et al. Effects of atorvastatin on early recurrent ischemic events in acute coronary syndromes: The MIRACL study: A randomized controlled trial. *JAMA.* 2001;285(13):1711–1718.
11. Antman EM, Cohen M, Bernink PJ, et al. The TIMI risk score for unstable angina/non-ST elevation MI: A method for prognostication and therapeutic decision making. *JAMA.* 2000;284(7):835–842.
12. Effectiveness of intravenous thrombolytic treatment in acute myocardial infarction. Gruppo Italiano per lo Studio della Streptochinasi nell'Infarto Miocardico (GISSI). *Lancet.* 1986;1(8478):397–402.
13. Randomised trial of intravenous streptokinase, oral aspirin, both, or neither among 17,187 cases of suspected acute myocardial infarction: ISIS-2. ISIS-2 (Second International Study of Infarct Survival) Collaborative Group. *Lancet.* 1988;2(8607):349–360.
14. Weaver WD, Simes RJ, Betriu A, et al. Comparison of primary coronary angioplasty and intravenous thrombolytic therapy for acute myocardial infarction: A quantitative review. *JAMA.* 1997;278(23):2093–2098.
15. Andersen HR, Nielsen TT, Rasmussen K, et al. A comparison of coronary angioplasty with fibrinolytic therapy in acute myocardial infarction. *N Engl J Med.* 2003;349(8):733–742.

16. Valgimigli M, Percoco G, Malagutti P, et al. Tirofiban and sirolimus-eluting stent vs abciximab and bare-metal stent for acute myocardial infarction: A randomized trial. *JAMA.* 2005;293(17):2109–2117.
17. Bavry AA, Kumbhani DJ, Rassi AN, et al. Benefit of early invasive therapy in acute coronary syndromes: A meta-analysis of contemporary randomized clinical trials. *J Am Coll Cardiol.* 2006;48(7):1319–1325.
18. Mehta SR, Cannon CP, Fox KAA, et al. Routine vs selective invasive strategies in patients with acute coronary syndromes: A collaborative meta-analysis of randomized trials. *JAMA.* 2005;293(23):2908–2917.
19. de Winter RJ, Windhausen F, Cornel JH, et al. Early invasive versus selectively invasive management for acute coronary syndromes. *N Engl J Med.* 2005;353(11):1095–1104.
20. Risk of myocardial infarction and death during treatment with low dose aspirin and intravenous heparin in men with unstable coronary artery disease. The RISC Group. *Lancet.* 1990;336(8719):827–830.
21. Eikelboom JW, Anand SS, Malmberg K, et al. Unfractionated heparin and low-molecular-weight heparin in acute coronary syndrome without ST elevation: A meta-analysis. *Lancet.* 2000;355(9219): 1936–1942.
22. Goodman SG, Fitchett D, Armstrong PW, et al. Randomized evaluation of the safety and efficacy of enoxaparin versus unfractionated heparin in high-risk patients with non-ST-segment elevation acute coronary syndromes receiving the glycoprotein IIb/IIIa inhibitor eptifibatide. *Circulation.* 2003;107(2):238–244.
23. Mehta SR, Yusuf S, Peters RJ, et al. Effects of pretreatment with clopidogrel and aspirin followed by long-term therapy in patients undergoing percutaneous coronary intervention: The PCI-CURE study. *Lancet.* 2001;358(9281):527–533.
24. Steinhubl SR, Berger PB, Mann JT, et al. Early and sustained dual oral antiplatelet therapy following percutaneous coronary intervention: A randomized controlled trial. *JAMA.* 2002;288(19):2411–2420.
25. Sabatine MS, Cannon CP, Gibson CM, et al. Effect of clopidogrel pretreatment before percutaneous coronary intervention in patients with ST-elevation myocardial infarction treated with fibrinolytics: The PCI-CLARITY study. *JAMA.* 2005;294(10):1224–1232.
26. Montalescot G, Barragan P, Wittenberg O, et al. Platelet glycoprotein IIb/IIIa inhibition with coronary stenting for acute myocardial infarction. *N Engl J Med.* 2001;344(25):1895–1903.
27. Boersma E, Harrington RA, Moliterno DJ, et al. Platelet glycoprotein IIb/IIIa inhibitors in acute coronary syndromes: A meta-analysis of all major randomised clinical trials. *Lancet.* 2002;359(9302):189–198.
28. Roffi M, Chew DP, Mukherjee D, et al. Platelet glycoprotein IIb/IIIa inhibitors reduce mortality in diabetic patients with non-ST-segment-elevation acute coronary syndromes. *Circulation.* 2001;104(23):2767–2771.

29. Hjalmarson A, Elmfeldt D, Herlitz J, et al. Effect on mortality of metoprolol in acute myocardial infarction. A double-blind randomised trial. *Lancet*. 1981;2(8251):823–827.

30. Randomised trial of intravenous atenolol among 16,027 cases of suspected acute myocardial infarction: ISIS-1. First International Study of Infarct Survival Collaborative Group. *Lancet*. 1986;2(8498): 57–66.

31. Roberts R, Rogers WJ, Mueller HS, et al. Immediate versus deferred beta-blockade following thrombolytic therapy in patients with acute myocardial infarction. Results of the Thrombolysis in Myocardial Infarction (TIMI) II-B Study. *Circulation*. 1991;83(2):422–437.

32. Chen ZM, Pan HC, Chen YP, et al. Early intravenous then oral metoprolol in 45,852 patients with acute myocardial infarction: Randomised placebo-controlled trial. *Lancet*. 2005;366(9497):1622–1632.

33. Dargie HJ. Effect of carvedilol on outcome after myocardial infarction in patients with left-ventricular dysfunction: The CAPRICORN randomised trial. *Lancet*. 2001;357(9266):1385–1390.

34. Randomised trial of cholesterol lowering in 4444 patients with coronary heart disease: The Scandinavian Simvastatin Survival Study (4S). *Lancet*. 1994;344(8934):1383–1389.

35. LaRosa JC, Grundy SM, Waters DD, et al. Intensive lipid lowering with atorvastatin in patients with stable coronary disease. *N Engl J Med*. 2005;352(14):1425–1435.

36. Cannon CP, Braunwald E, McCabe CH, et al. Intensive versus moderate lipid lowering with statins after acute coronary syndromes. *N Engl J Med*. 2004;350(15):1495–1504.

37. Pfeffer MA, Braunwald E, Moyé LA, et al. Effect of captopril on mortality and morbidity in patients with left ventricular dysfunction after myocardial infarction. Results of the survival and ventricular enlargement trial. The SAVE Investigators. *N Engl J Med*. 1992;327(10):669–677.

38. Ambrosioni E, Borghi C, Magnani B. The effect of the angiotensin-converting-enzyme inhibitor zofenopril on mortality and morbidity after anterior myocardial infarction. The Survival of Myocardial Infarction Long-Term Evaluation (SMILE) Study Investigators. *N Engl J Med*. 1995;332(2):80–85.

39. Effect of ramipril on mortality and morbidity of survivors of acute myocardial infarction with clinical evidence of heart failure. The Acute Infarction Ramipril Efficacy (AIRE) Study Investigators. *Lancet*. 1993;342(8875):821–828.

40. Pitt B, Remme W, Zannad F, et al. Eplerenone, a selective aldosterone blocker, in patients with left ventricular dysfunction after myocardial infarction. *N Engl J Med*. 2003;348(14):1309–1321.

CHAPTER 4

Cardiogenic Shock

DAVID V. DANIELS, TODD J. BRINTON,
AND RANDALL VAGELOS

BACKGROUND

Cardiogenic shock is a state of inadequate tissue perfusion and dysoxia due to primary cardiac dysfunction clinically manifest by systemic hypotension and end-organ compromise.

* Historical mortality approaches 80% without revascularization[1]
* Current era mortality remains as high as 60%[2]
* Complicates 7%–9% of all acute myocardial infarctions (AMI)[3,4]
* Shock criteria often absent on admission (<10% of patients) but usually develops early in the hospitalization (mean time MI to onset 5.5 hours in the SHOCK trial registry)
* Multifactorial etiologies (LV failure – 79%, Severe MR – 7%, acute ventricular septal defect (VSD) – 4%, isolated right ventricular (RV) failure – 2%, tamponade – 1.4%[2])
* Majority of cases secondary to AMI present with ST segment elevation myocardial infarct (STEMI)

FEATURES OF CARDIOGENIC SHOCK[5]

* Persistent systemic hypotension: systolic blood pressure (SBP) <90 mm Hg or mean arterial pressure (MAP) >30 mm Hg below baseline
* Cardiac index <1.8 liters/min/m^2 or inotrope dependence to maintain cardiac output and blood pressure (BP)
* Pulmonary artery wedge pressure (PAWP) >18 mm Hg
* Signs of systemic hypoperfusion (cool extremities, oliguria, lactic acidosis)

HISTORY

* Rapid diagnosis essential: history and physical exam should be focused and brief with simultaneous initial resuscitation
* Inquire about time course of symptoms, new or changing angina, shortness of breath (SOB), paroxysmal nocturnal dyspnea (PND), orthopnea, edema, weight changes, or fatigue

- History of MI, heart failure (HF), or valvular disease
- Recent changes in medication dose or type

PHYSICAL EXAM

Look for the following:
- Absolute or relative hypotension (SBP >30 mm Hg below baseline)
- Check bilateral blood pressures if hypotension suspected as unilateral subclavian or axillary stenosis may falsely classify patients as centrally hypotensive.
- Narrow pulse pressure (pulse pressure <25% of the SBP has a sensitivity and specificity of 91% and 83% for a cardiac index of <2.2 L/min/m^2)[4]
- Cool underperfused extremities, altered mental status, low urine output
- Pulmonary edema and respiratory distress
- Signs of HF: Elevated JVP, S3, S4, tachycardia, hypoxia, crackles
- Peripheral edema suggests some component of chronic HF and can be absent with acute HF
- New systolic murmur suggests acute mitral regurgitation (MR) or VSD, assess for a thrill
- Listen with patient leaning forward to detect the diastolic murmur of AI
- Asymmetric pulses and a focal neurologic exam (aortic dissection)

LABORATORY EXAMS AND IMAGING

Labs
- Complete blood count (CBC) w/ diff, comprehensive metabolic panel (CMP), cardiac enzymes, APTT/PT, BNP
- Serial lactate measurements and ABGs useful in following tissue perfusion and response to therapy

ECG
- Rapid assessment of potential acute coronary syndrome (ACS), arrhythmia, or heart block
- Although most ACS associated with cardiogenic shock presents as a STEMI, significant ST depression or other signs of ischemia should prompt consideration of early angiography in the setting of shock
- Inferior ST elevation should prompt R sided leads to assess for RV injury or infarct
- Isolated anterior ST depression should prompt posterior leads to assess for true posterior STEMI

Chest X-ray
- Assess mediastinum and always consider aortic dissection

- Pulmonary edema (1/3 of patients *without* pulmonary edema in the SHOCK trial)
- Clear lungs with hypotension +/− hypoxia, consider massive PE

Echo
- An extremely useful test for systolic function, regional WMAs, RV infarct, mechanical complications of MI, tamponade, and valvular lesions
- Transesophageal echocardiography (TEE) may be necessary for technically suboptimal transthoracic echocardiogram (TTE), on ventilator, or to evaluate for aortic dissection (especially in unstable patients who can't go to computed tomography (CT))

Helical CT of the Chest
- Useful to assess for proximal pulmonary embollism (PE) and aortic dissection (sensitivity only 83% for proximal dissection in one study)
- Sensitivity and specificity probably institutional and reader dependent
- Even if patient is in acute renal failure (ARF) the benefits of IV contrast likely outweigh the risks in this patient population and may need to consider dialysis
- Different phase of contrast needed for optimal PE and aortic dissection evaluations

TABLE 4-1	Etiology of cardiogenic shock
Etiology	**Findings**
Acute severe LV failure (most common cause of cardiogenic shock)	– Often from massive anterior infarct – ST elevation often seen – Consider in aggressive titration of HF meds → decompensation
Mechanical complications of AMI	Papillary muscle rupture or dysfunction w/ severe MR – Classically 2–7 days post-MI – More common with inferior/posterior infarct because of single blood supply to posterior papillary muscle via the RCA – Often with an early systolic murmur vs. classic holosystolic murmur because of early systolic equalization of LV → LA pressure – Echo with severe MR, +/− flail leaflet Acute ventricular septal defect (vsd) – Higher risk with "wrap around LAD" should be alerted to this complication when anterior STEMI presents with concomitant inferior lead ST elevation (OR 17)[8] – Anterior MI → apical VSD – Inferior MI → basal VSD – Holosystolic murmur radiating to R sternal border often with a thrill

(continued)

TABLE 4-1 *(Continued)*

Etiology	Findings
	− PO_2 step-up from RA to RV/PA (use the swan that's in!) − Echo dx by color Doppler cardiac tamponade (free wall rupture or hemorrhagic effusion) − Beck's triad: hypotension, distant heart sounds, JVD − Pulsus paradoxus − Echo support of dx by effusion + RA/RV diastolic collapse, PW Doppler − Swan: Equalization of diastolic pressures − RA = RVD = PAD Can see as an early complication of PCI (coronary rupture)
RV infarct	− Seen most often with concomitant inferior wall MI − Check R sided leads − JVD, + Kussmaul's sign, hypotensive response to NTG and diuretics, responds to fluids, generally clear lungs − May see bradycardia, heart block, GI symptoms from RCA ACS − Echo will show RV dilation, hypokinesis − Swan: RA pressure >10 mm Hg and RA:PCWP >0.8
Stress cardiomyopathy (Tako tsubo) Or "broken heart syndrome"	− Consider as a cause of cardiogenic shock in ST elevation with normal epicardial coronary arteries − Preponderance of post menopausal females, often significant "life stressor" is identifiable − Look for apical or more rarely basal ballooning − Consider acute LVOT obstruction as an etiology of shock; if present, trial of phenylephrine
RV failure secondary to massive PE	− Signs and symptoms of acute RV failure in the absence of AMI − Echo with dilated RV − Diagnosis by Helical CT angiography
Proximal aortic dissection	− Pulse deficits and focal neuro exam − Suspect with widened mediastinum on CXR − Severe AI with extension to the root on Echo − Cardiac tamponade − May see inferior STEMI because the RCA is most often compromised by dissection
Tachyarrhythmias	− AF/Atrial flutter w/ RVR, VT
Bradyarrhythmias	− Anterior infarct → Mobitz II or CHB with slow ventricular escape − Inferior infarct → sinus bradycardia, Mobitz I → CHB usually with junctional escape
Myocarditis	− Acute LV dysfunction, positive enzymes, +/− fever and viral prodrome
Endocarditis	− Acute valvular regurgitation in the setting of septic picture and vegetations − Positive blood cultures

Etiology	Findings
Hemorrhagic shock	– Either as a primary presentation or as a complication of thrombolytics and anticoagulants – Shock with low filling pressures
Septic shock	– Can see LV dysfunction in severe sepsis – Can see positive cardiac enzymes

LV, left ventricular; LAD, left anterior descending; LVOT, left ventricular outfloor tract.

INITIAL EVALUATION AND TREATMENT

See Figure 4-1 and Table 4-1.

SPECIFIC THERAPIES

Antithrombotic Therapy and Anticoagulation

- Patients with STEMI or ACS should be treated with ASA, heparin, GPIIB/IIIA inhibitors (see chapter on CP and ACS)
- Strongly consider withholding Clopidogrel if early angiography planned and patient is a surgical candidate (lack of comorbidities and multiorgan system disease) as up to 40% of patients may benefit from emergent CABG and bleeding may complicate an already critically ill patient
- Retrospective subgroup data from PURSUIT suggests benefit of eptifibatide in cardiogenic shock complicating non-ST elevation ACS (NSTE ACS)[5]
- Improvement in TIMI 3 flow with the use of GPIIB/IIIA inhibitors in TIGER-PA trial prior to PCI versus during would suggest improvements in microvascular obstruction as a possible mechanism[6]

Revascularization

- Associated with significant mortality benefit in AMI complicated by cardiogenic shock
- Timing of reperfusion is highly correlated with outcomes: 44% mortality if admitted within 3 hours from symptom onset versus 58% from 12–24 hours[7]
- TIMI flow grade of infarct related artery (IRA) highly correlated with mortality: 27% in IRAs with TIMI grade 3 flow versus 47% with TIMI grade 0/1 flow[8]
- In the landmark, "SHould we emergently revascularize Occluded Coronaries for cardiogenic shocK" (SHOCK) randomized trial, successful angioplasty (TIMI grade 2 or 3 flow) associated with 38% 30 day mortality versus 79% in unsuccessful angioplasty (TIMI grade 0 or 1 flow), lending support to the open artery hypothesis[9]

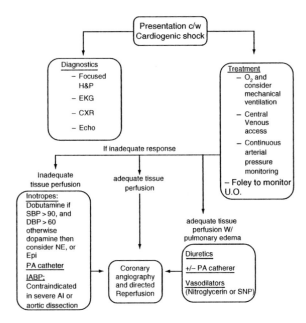

FIGURE 4-1 Initial evaluation and treatment of cardiogenic shock. Markers of poor tissue perfusion include altered mentation, oliguria, cool extremities, azotemia, and lactic acidosis.

Initial Medical Therapy versus Emergent Revascularization

- SHOCK trial *mortality* 50% with emergent revascularization (60% PCI, 40% CABG) versus 63% at 6 months with initial medical therapy and subsequent targeted revascularization[9]
- Number needed to treat of eight to prevent one death
- Benefit is probably beyond thrombolysis as 63% of initial medical therapy group and 49% of revascularization group got thrombolytic therapy
- More benefit in those <75 years old
- Sustained benefits at 6 years[6]

Thrombolysis + IABP

- Suggestion of mortality benefit with thrombolytic therapy (TT) in post-hoc analysis of the SHOCK trial in the medical treatment group 60% mortality with versus 78% without TT though assignment to TT was not randomized and results may represent selection bias[10]
- Strongly consider IABP placement by an experienced operator as substantial mortality benefit with the use of an IABP + TT,[11] and there is NO proven benefit with TT alone (see Figure 4-2)

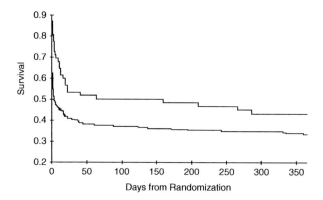

FIGURE 4-2 Effect of IABP added to thrombolysis on mortality in cardiogenic shock (GUSTO I, JACC 1997).

* Given high rate of thrombolysis in the early revascularization arm of SHOCK (and lack of harm), it is reasonable to employ a strategy of IABP placement and thrombolysis followed by emergent transfer to a facility capable of PCI if such a transfer is likely to be delayed >90 minutes

Percutaneous Ventricular Assist Device (PVAD)—Tandem Heart

* Placed in the cath lab with a left atrial inflow catheter (via transseptal puncture) and a femoral artery return catheter
* Initial study in cardiogenic shock showed improvement of cardiac index from 1.7 → 2.4 L/m/m^2 and significant improvements in CVP and PCWP[12]
* Randomized trial of PVAD versus intra-aortic balloon pump (IABP) revealed improvement in hemodynamic parameters in the PVAD group but with higher bleeding and leg ischemia complications and no difference in mortality[13]
* Can consider PVAD as an aggressive support intervention if IABP support is inadequate in the setting of refractory cardiogenic shock

REFERENCES

1. Holmes DR, Berger PB, Hochman JS, et al. Cardiogenic shock in patients with acute ischemic syndromes with and without ST-segment elevation. *Circulation*. 1999;100(20):2067–2073.
2. Hochman JS, Buller CE, Sleeper LA, et al. Cardiogenic shock complicating acute myocardial infarction—etiologies, management and

outcome: A report from the SHOCK Trial Registry. Should we emergently revascularize Occluded Coronaries for cardiogenic shocK? *J Am Coll Cardiol.* 2000;36(3 Suppl A):1063–1070.

3. Stevenson LW, Perloff JK. The limited reliability of physical signs for estimating hemodynamics in chronic heart failure. *JAMA.* 1989;261(6):884–888.

4. Hasdai D, Harrington RA, Hochman JS, et al. Platelet glycoprotein IIb/IIIa blockade and outcome of cardiogenic shock complicating acute coronary syndromes without persistent ST-segment elevation. *J Am Coll Cardiol.* 2000;36(3): 685–692.

5. Fuster V, Alexander RW, O'Rourke RA. *Hurst's the Heart.* 11th ed. New York: McGraw-Hill Medical Publishing Division; 2004.

6. Hochman JS, Sleeper LA, Webb JG, et al. Early revascularization and long-term survival in cardiogenic shock complicating acute myocardial infarction. *JAMA.* 2006;295(21):2511–2515.

7. Zeymer U, Vogt A, Zahn R, et al. Predictors of in-hospital mortality in 1333 patients with acute myocardial infarction complicated by cardiogenic shock treated with primary percutaneous coronary intervention (PCI): Results of the primary PCI registry of the Arbeitsgemeinschaft Leitende Kardiologische Krankenhausärzte (ALKK). *Eur Heart J.* 2004;25(4):322–328.

8. Wong SC, Sanborn T, Sleeper LA, et al. Angiographic findings and clinical correlates in patients with cardiogenic shock complicating acute myocardial infarction: A report from the SHOCK Trial Registry. SHould we emergently revascularize Occluded Coronaries for cardiogenic shocK? *J Am Coll Cardiol.* 2000;36(3 Suppl A):1077–1083.

9. Hochman JS, Sleeper LA, Webb JG, et al. Early revascularization in acute myocardial infarction complicated by cardiogenic shock. SHOCK Investigators. Should we emergently revascularize occluded coronaries for cardiogenic shock? *N Engl J Med.* 1999;341(9):625–634.

10. French JK, Feldman HA, Assmann SF, et al. Influence of thrombolytic therapy, with or without intra-aortic balloon counterpulsation, on 12-month survival in the SHOCK trial. *Am Heart J.* 2003;146(5):804–810.

11. Hayashi T, Hirano Y, Takai H, et al. Usefulness of ST-segment elevation in the inferior leads in predicting ventricular septal rupture in patients with anterior wall acute myocardial infarction. *Am J Cardiol.* 2005;96(8):1037–1041.

12. Thiele H, Lauer B, Hambrecht R, et al. Reversal of cardiogenic shock by percutaneous left atrial-to-femoral arterial bypass assistance. *Circulation.* 2001;104(24):2917–2922.

13. Thiele H, Sick P, Boudriot E, et al. Randomized comparison of intra-aortic balloon support with a percutaneous left ventricular assist device in patients with revascularized acute myocardial infarction complicated by cardiogenic shock. *Eur Heart J.* 2005;26(13):1276–1283.

CHAPTER 5

Bradyarrhythmias and Pacing

JAMES V. FREEMAN AND PAUL J. WANG

BACKGROUND

Bradyarrhythmias result from abnormalities of sinus node function or A-V conduction. In this chapter we review the initial recognition, triage, acute management, and definitive therapy for the bradyarrhythmias.

DEFINITIONS

Bradycardia

Bradycardia is defined as a ventricular heart rate <60 beats per minute (bpm), and sinus bradycardia exists when each QRS complex is preceded by a P wave of sinus node origin on the electrocardiogram (ECG).

Sinus Node Dysfunction

Sinoatrial blocks: Sinoatrial (S-A) blocks are uncommon and occur when there is disturbance of the conduction of the electrical impulse from the heart's normal pacemaker, the S-A node, to the surrounding atrium. (See Figure 5-1.) The severity of dysfunction can vary widely and there are many ECG findings associated with S-A blocks (also called S-A exit blocks).[1] The S-A blocks can be categorized as first, second, and third degree based on the characteristics of the conduction disturbance.

First Degree

In first-degree S-A block, there is an increased time for the S-A node's impulse to reach and depolarize the rest of the atrium and form a P wave on ECG (Figure 5-1). There are no abnormalities seen on the 12-lead tracing with first-degree S-A block because impulse origination from the S-A node still produces a normal P wave on the 12-lead ECG.[2]

70

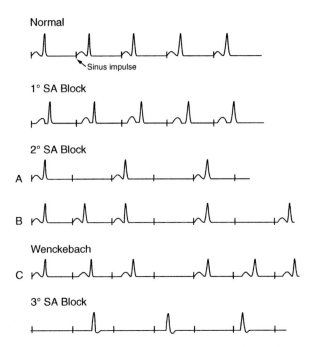

FIGURE 5-1 Sinoatrial (S-A) block. Normal sinus rhythms with various degrees of S-A block. Sinus impulses not seen on the body surface ECG are represented by the vertical lines. With first-degree S-A block, although there is prolongation of the interval between the sinus impulses and the P wave, such a delay cannot be detected on the ECG. A: Persistent 2:1 S-A block cannot be distinguished from marked sinus bradycardia. B: The diagnosis of second-degree S-A block depends on the presence of pause or pauses that are the multiple of the basic P-P interval. C: When there is a Wenckebach phenomenon, there is gradual shortening of the P-P interval before the pause. With third-degree S-A block, the ECG records only the escape rhythm. (Used with permission from Suawicz B, Knilans TK. *Chou's electrocardiography in clinical practice.* 5th ed. Philadelphia: WB Saunders; 2001:321.)

Second Degree

Type I (Wenckebach): In second-degree S-A block type I, there is a progressively increasing interval for each S-A nodal impulse to depolarize the atrial myocardium and produce a P wave on ECG (Figure 5-1). This interval continues to lengthen until the S-A node's impulse does not depolarize the atrium at all, which is manifested on ECG by a gradual shortening of the P-P interval with an eventual dropping of a P wave. It can be recognized by grouped beatings of the P waves, with sinus pauses.

Type II: In second-degree S-A block type II, there is a fixed interval between the S-A node impulse and the depolarization of the atrium with an intermittent S-A nodal impulse that fails to conduct to the atrium (Figure 5-1). This manifests on ECG as a dropped P wave with a P-P interval surrounding the pause that is two to four times the length of the baseline P-P interval.[3]

Second-degree S-A Block with 2:1 Conduction

In second-degree S-A block with 2:1 conduction, every other impulse from the S-A node causes atrial depolarization while the other is dropped. It is impossible to differentiate this from sinus bradycardia on ECG unless the beginning or termination of the S-A block is recorded, in which case it manifests as a distinct halving (beginning) or doubling (termination) of the baseline heart rate.

Third Degree

In third-degree S-A block, none of the S-A nodal impulses depolarize the atrium, which appears on ECG as either atrial stand-still or P waves retrogradely conducted from a junctional rhythm (Figure 5-1). Sometimes there can be a long pause on the ECG until a normal sinus rhythm is resumed, which can be difficult to distinguish from sinus pause or arrest due to abnormalities of sinus impulse formation.

Sinus pause/sinus arrest: Sinus pause and sinus arrest are characterized by the failure of the S-A node to form an impulse, manifesting on the ECG as a sinus pause of varying length.[1] Some sinus pauses follow the spontaneous termination of atrial fibrillation because of the overdrive suppression of the sinus node.

Sick sinus syndrome: Sick sinus syndrome includes a range of S-A node dysfunction that includes inappropriate sinus bradycardia, sinus arrhythmia, sinus pause/arrest, S-A block, A-V junctional (escape) rhythm, and the tachycardia-bradycardia syndrome (covered in the tachyarrhythmias chapter).[4]

Atrioventricular Conduction Dysfunction

Atrioventricular block: In atrioventricular block, electrical conduction is disturbed between the atrium and the ventricle. As with S-A blocks, A-V blocks are categorized into first-, second-, and third-degree blocks based on the characteristics of the conduction disturbance.

First Degree

First-degree A-V block is defined as a prolonged P-R interval, greater than 200 milliseconds, which remains constant. (See Figure 5-2.) On ECG, the P wave and QRS complex have normal morphology, and a P wave precedes each QRS complex. The lengthening of the P-R interval results from a conduction delay from within the atrium, the A-V node, or the His-Purkinje system.

Second Degree

Mobitz Type I (Wenckebach): Second-degree A-V block Mobitz type I is characterized by a P-R interval that lengthens progressively until an impulse fails to conduct to the ventricles and a QRS complex is dropped. (See Figure 5-3.) This block usually occurs at the level of the A-V node and above the His bundle. The patient's QRS complex is usually narrow (less than or equal to 120 milliseconds) although there may be a concomitant lower conduction disturbance leading to bundle branch block. On ECG, the P-R interval lengthens as the R-R interval shortens, and the R-R interval that contains the dropped beat is less than the sum of two of the shortest R-R intervals seen on the ECG. Also, on the ECG rhythm strip, a grouping of beats can be seen.[2,7] A consistent and diagnostic feature of Wenkebach is that the PR interval after the dropped beat is shorter than those immediately preceding the AV block.

Mobitz Type II: Second-degree A-V block Mobitz type II is defined by a constant P-R interval that may be normal or prolonged (>0.20 s) and periodic abrupt failure of the atrial impulse to conduct to the ventricles. (See Figure 5-4.) The QRS complex is nearly always widened, since development of Mobitz Type II block almost always follows development of bundle branch block. This rule is so strong that apparently abrupt A-V block without measurable preceding P-R prolongation in a patient with a narrow QRS complex

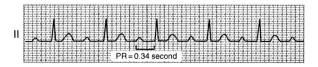

FIGURE 5-2 First degree AV block: The PR interval here is > 200 ms with a 1:1 relationship of P waves to QRS complexes. (With permission: Goldberger: *Clinical Electrocardiography: A Simplified Approach*. 2006, Mosby.)

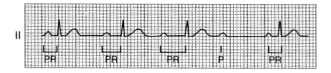

FIGURE 5-3 Mobitz Type I (Wenkebach) Second degree AV block: Fixed P-P interval with progressive PR prolongation with development of AV block. Note the PR interval on the beat after the pause is the shortest which is diagnostic of Wenkebach. (With permission: Goldberger: *Clinical Electrocardiography: A Simplified Approach.* 2006, Mosby.)

is more likely to be at the level of the A-V node and thus be an atypical Mobitz Type I A-V block rather than actually representing Mobitz Type II A-V block.

Second-degree A-V block with 2:1 conduction: In second-degree A-V block with 2:1 conduction, every other QRS complex is dropped, causing two P waves for each QRS complex. Since there is no way to determine on ECG if the P-R interval lengthens before the dropped QRS complex, the primary method of determining the level of the block is examining the QRS width. If the QRS complex is narrow, the 2:1 A-V block almost certainly exists at the level of the A-V node. If the QRS complex is widened, the level of the block could be either at the level of the A-V node or infrahisian.

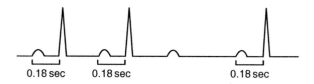

FIGURE 5-4 Second degree type II AV block: Fixed P-P interval with fixed PR interval and development of AV block. Note the PR interval on the beat after the pause is identical to the one prior. This is in contradistinction to Wenkebach. (With permission: Goldberger: *Clinical Electrocardiography: A Simplified Approach.* 2006, Mosby.)

Third Degree

Third-degree A-V block, or complete heart block, occurs when no electrical impulses from the atria conduct through to the ventricles. (See Figure 5-5.) The atria and ventricles thus depolarize and beat independently. An escape rhythm originating from the A-V junction or the ventricles below the level of the block maintains the ventricular rate. In third-degree A-V block, the P waves march out regularly and independently of the regular ventricular depolarization (QRS complexes). The atrial rate is generally faster than the ventricular rate, because the latter is an escape rhythm, and the ventricular rate can vary depending upon where the ventricular depolarization originates.[1] In some cases, the P-P interval encompassing the escape QRS complex may be shorter than otherwise in the tracing, a phenomenon called "ventriculophasic phenomenon."

Escape Rhythms

When electrical impulses fail to conduct to the ventricles from the atria, whether due to S-A block or A-V block, ventricular depolarization can originate from more distal locations in the conduction system that also possess automaticity. Generally the more distal the site of impulse origination, the slower the rate generated. The ventricular rate is generally 40 to 60 bpm with a narrow QRS complex when it is driven by a junctional pacemaker within the A-V node or above the His bundle. A ventricular pacemaker is characterized by a widened QRS and a rate less than 40 bpm (except an accelerated idioventricular rhythm with a rate > 40 bpm). These rhythms originate in the His-Purkinje system and are usually associated with a poorer prognosis.[7] If no escape impulse is generated, then the result is an asystolic arrest.

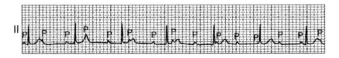

FIGURE 5-5 Third degree (Complete) AV block: Fixed P-P interval with AV dissociation: No relationship between P waves and the QRS complexes. In this case the escape pacemaker is junctional and hence the QRS is narrow and rate is relatively faster than a ventricular escape. (With permission: Goldberger: *Clinical Electrocardiography: A Simplified Approach.* 2006, Mosby.)

CAUSES

Intrinsic abnormalities of conduction may occur as the result of many complex changes in the cardiac conduction system:

- Congenital
  - Related to maternal lupus
  - Related to congenital heart disease
  - L-transposition of the great arteries
- Genetic abnormalities
- Immunologic
  - Lyme disease
- Infectious
  - Endocarditis
  - Lyme disease
- Idiopathic degeneration and fibrosis
- Ischemia or infarction
- Infiltrative diseases
  - Sarcoidosis
  - Amyloidosis
- Trauma
  - During valve replacement surgery
  - During radiofrequency catheter ablation
  - Extra-cardiac causes:
    - Electrolyte abnormalities
    - Hypothyroidism
    - Hypothermia
    - Increased intracranial pressure
    - Vasovagal reactions
    - Drugs, for example: lithium, amiodarone, digoxin, beta-adrenergic receptor antagonists, calcium channel antagonists[9]

CLINICAL PRESENTATIONS

Bradycardia can result in cerebral hypoperfusion leading to symptoms such as presyncope, syncope, confusion, memory loss, and, rarely, seizure activity. Inability of the heart rate to increase in response to increased physiologic demand, called chronotropic incompetence, can occur even when true bradycardia is not present and can result in subjective effort intolerance, fatigue, weakness, and dyspnea.[10] Sometimes, patients with advanced A-V block appear to be asymptomatic. Patients with sinus node dysfunction and atrial arrhythmias, the tachycardia-bradycardia syndrome, can present with complaints of palpitations as well as symptoms related to bradycardia.

It is extremely important to take a careful medication history with particular focus on medications that may impair sinus node and A-V nodal function.

PHYSICAL EXAM

- Bradycardia, regular or irregular, depending on specific arrhythmia
- Systemic hypotension in the absence of concomitant vasodilation or vasodepressor phenomenon may not be present; the systolic pressure generated after a pause may be higher than the average systolic blood pressure
- Evidence of impaired alertness or cognitive function may be due to cerebral hypoperfusion
- If some P waves are blocked, there will be a lack of coordination of the A wave in the jugular venous waves with the carotid impulse. With complete A-V block or prolongation of the P-R interval to more than 300 milliseconds, asynchronous atrial and ventricular contraction can result in cannon A waves.
- Pulmonary congestion, and in severe cases peripheral
- Typical rash of Lyme disease
- Manifestations of underlying congenital heart disease or cardiomyopathy such as murmurs or gallops

LAB EXAMS AND IMAGING

Lab

- Cardiac enzymes to rule out myocardial infarction or ischemia as the predisposing condition
- Electrolyte abnormalities
- BNP if there is evidence of heart failure
- Drug levels of agents such as digoxin, lithium, and anti-arrhythmics
- Thyroid function tests
- Lyme titers if Lyme disease is suspected
- Blood cultures if infection is suspected

Chest X-ray

- Examine lung fields for evidence of pulmonary congestion and abnormal chamber size

Echocardiogram

- Useful to evaluate for wall motion abnormalities, effusions, or valvular lesions secondary to ischemia/infarction, infiltrative process, and congenital abnormalities
- Evidence of cardiac vegetations due to endocarditis

MRI/CT

* May play a role in identifying areas of ischemia/infarction and in ruling out rare infiltrative processes such as amyloidosis or tumors

INITIAL MANAGEMENT

Initial management of patients with bradycardia should be directed at identifying and treating reversible causes and at providing rate support for those that are symptomatic. Temporary pacing is generally indicated in patients with symptomatic bradycardia that is likely to recur, particularly in the setting of syncope. Pacing may be performed initially transcutaneously, but this method is not well tolerated due to pain and is unreliable for prolonged

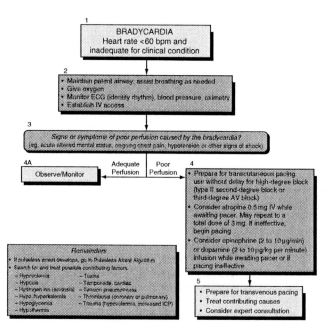

FIGURE 5-6 ACLS bradycardia treatment algorithm. (From 2005 American Heart Association Guidelines for Cardiopulmonary Resuscitation and Emergency Cardiovascular Care; Part 7.3: Management of Symptomatic Bradycardia and Tachycardia. *Circulation.* 2005;112: IV-67–IV-77.)

periods. Thus, transvenous pacing is generally preferred. For mild degrees of bradycardia, particularly in reversible settings, acutely, sinus bradycardia or A-V block with a narrow QRS complex may be treated with intravenous atropine, usually 0.5 to 1.0 mg. For a wide QRS complex, atropine may worsen the degree of A-V block since it may increase the sinus rate but not improve A-V block below the level of the His bundle. Isoproterenol or epinephrine is generally used in this setting. Figure 5-6 also indicates that IV dopamine may be used.

Oral theophylline has been used with some success in the treatment of sinus bradycardia that is likely to be transient.[11]

INDICATION FOR HOSPITALIZATION

All patients with a severe or symptomatic bradycardia should be admitted to a monitored setting to ensure prompt diagnosis and treatment. Patients who require temporary or permanent pacemaker therapy according to the American College of Cardiology/American Heart Association Task Force guidelines should be hospitalized for pacemaker implantation. (See Tables 5-1 through 5-4.) Patients should be admitted to the cardiac intensive care unit (CCU) or an intermediate cardiac care unit if the cause of the bradyarrhythmia necessitates admission (e.g., acute coronary syndrome), or if temporary pacemaker support is needed while awaiting definitive therapy.[10]

 TABLE 5-1 Common indications for temporary cardiac pacing

1. Therapeutically, for symptomatic bradycardia

    a. Persistent bradycardia, until permanent pacemaker implantation can be accomplished
    b. Transient bradycardia (e.g., acute myocardial infarction)

2. Prophylactically, for potential bradycardia that may produce symptoms or hemodynamic embarrassment in acute myocardial infarction

    a. New bundle-branch block
    b. New bi- or trifascicular block with first-degree A-V block
    c. Type I second-degree A-V block with wide QRS complexes at slow rate
    d. Type II second-degree A-V block or higher degrees of A-V block
    e. Prophylactically, to prevent pause-dependent ventricular tachyarrhythmias

Adapted from Hongo RH, Goldschlager NF. Bradycardia and pacemakers. In Wachter RM, Goldman L, Hollander H, eds. *Hospital Medicine.* 2nd ed. Philadelphia: Lippincott Williams & Wilkins. 2005.[10]

TABLE 5-2 — Indications for permanent pacing in sinus node dysfunction

Class I (conditions for which there is evidence and/or general agreement that a given procedure or treatment is useful and effective)

1. Sinus node dysfunction with documented symptomatic bradycardia, including frequent sinus pauses that produce symptoms; in some patients, bradycardia is iatrogenic and occurs as a consequence of essential long-term drug therapy of a type and dose for which there are no acceptable alternatives (Level of evidence C*)
2. Symptomatic chronotropic incompetence (Level of evidence C)

Class II (conditions for which there is conflicting evidence and/or divergence of opinion about the usefulness/efficacy of a procedure or treatment)

Class IIa (weight of evidence/opinion is in favor of usefulness/efficacy)

1. Sinus node dysfunction, occurring spontaneously or as a result of necessary drug therapy, with heart rate <40 bpm when a clear association between significant symptoms consistent with bradycardia and the actual presence of bradycardia has not been documented (Level of evidence C)
2. Syncope of unexplained origin when major abnormalities of sinus node function are discovered or provoked in electrophysiologic studies (Level of evidence C)

Class IIb (usefulness/efficacy is less well established by evidence/opinion)

1. In minimally symptomatic patients, chronic heart rate <40 bpm while awake (Level of evidence C)

Class III (conditions for which there is evidence and/or general agreement that a procedure/treatment is not useful/effective and in some cases may be harmful)

1. Sinus node dysfunction in asymptomatic patients, including those in whom substantial sinus bradycardia (heart rate <40 bpm) is a consequence of long-term drug treatment
2. Sinus node dysfunction in patients with symptoms suggestive of bradycardia and clearly documented as not associated with a slow heart rate
3. Sinus node dysfunction with symptomatic bradycardia due to nonessential drug therapy

*The weight of the evidence was ranked highest (A) if the data were derived from multiple randomized clinical trials that involved large numbers of patients and intermediate (B) if the data were derived from a limited number of randomized trials that involved small numbers of patients or from careful analyses of nonrandomized studies or observational registries. A lower rank (C) was given when expert opinion was the primary basis for the recommendation.

Adapted with permission from Gregoratos G, Abrams J, Epstein AE, et al. ACC/AHA/NASPE 2002 guideline update for implantation of cardiac pacemakers and antiarrhythmia devices—summary article. *J Am Coll Cardiol.* 2002;40:1703–1719. Copyright 2002 by the American College of Cardiology and American Heart Association, Inc.[13]

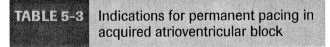

TABLE 5-3 Indications for permanent pacing in acquired atrioventricular block

Class I

1. Third-degree and advanced second-degree A-V block at any anatomic level, associated with any one of the following conditions:
   a. Bradycardia with symptoms (including heart failure) presumed to be due to A-V block (Level of evidence C)
   b. Arrhythmias and other medical conditions that require drugs that result in symptomatic bradycardia (Level of evidence C)
   c. Documented periods of asystole ≥3.0 s or any escape rate <40 bpm in awake, symptom-free patients (Level of evidence B, C)
   d. After catheter ablation of the A-V junction
   e. Postoperative A-V block that is not expected to resolve after cardiac surgery (Level of evidence C)
   f. Neuromuscular diseases with A-V block (e.g., myotonic muscular dystrophy, Kearns-Sayre syndrome, Erb limb-girdle dystrophy, and peroneal muscular atrophy) with or without symptoms, because there may be unpredictable progression of A-V conduction disease (Level of evidence B)
2. Second-degree A-V block with associated symptomatic bradycardia, regardless of the type or site of block (Level of evidence B)

Class IIa

1. Asymptomatic third-degree A-V block at any anatomic site with average awake ventricular rates of >40 bpm, especially if cardiomegaly or left ventricular dysfunction is present (Level of evidence B, C)
2. Asymptomatic type II second-degree A-V block with narrow QRS; when type II second-degree A-V block occurs with a wide QRS, pacing becomes a Class I recommendation (Level of evidence B)
3. Asymptomatic type I second-degree A-V block at intra- or infra-His levels found at electrophysiologic study performed for other indications (Level of evidence B)
4. First- or second-degree A-V block with symptoms similar to those of *pacemaker syndrome* (Level of evidence B)

Class IIb

1. Marked first-degree A-V block (>0.30 s) in patients with left ventricular dysfunction and symptoms of congestive heart failure in whom a shorter A-V interval results in hemodynamic improvement (Level of evidence C)
2. Neuromuscular disease (e.g., myotonic muscular dystrophy, Kearns-Sayre syndrome, Erb limb-girdle dystrophy, and peroneal muscular atrophy) with any degree of A-V block (including first-degree A-V block) with or without symptoms, because there may be unpredictable progression of A-V conduction disease (Level of evidence B)

Class III

1. Asymptomatic first-degree A-V block (Level of evidence B)
2. Asymptomatic type I second-degree A-V block at the supra-His (A-V node) level or not known to be intra- or infra-Hisian (Level of evidence B, C)

3. A-V block expected to resolve and/or unlikely to recur (e.g., drug toxicity, Lyme disease, or during hypoxia in sleep apnea syndrome in absence of symptoms) (Level of evidence B)

See Table 5-2 for definitions of classes and levels of evidence.

[a] A symptom complex of fatigue, weakness, dizziness, hypotension, effort intolerance, and pulmonary and central venous hypertension caused by inappropriate relationships between atrial and ventricular depolarization-contraction sequences.

Adapted with permission from Gregoratos G, Abrams J, Epstein AE, et al. ACC/AHA/NASPE 2002 guideline update for implantation of cardiac pacemakers and antiarrhythmia devices—summary article. *J Am Coll Cardiol.* 2002;40:1703–1719. Copyright 2002 by the American College of Cardiology and American Heart Association, Inc.[13]

 TABLE 5-4 Indications for permanent pacing after the acute phase of a myocardial infarction

Class I

1. Persistent second-degree A-V block in the His-Purkinje system with bilateral bundle-branch block or third-degree A-V block within or below the His-Purkinje system (Level of evidence B)
2. Transient advanced (second- or third-degree) infranodal A-V block and associated bundle-branch block; if the block site is uncertain, an electrophysiologic study may be necessary (Level of evidence B)
3. Persistent and symptomatic second- or third-degree A-V block (Level of evidence B)

Class IIa
None

Class IIb

1. Persistent second- or third-degree A-V block at the A-V node level (Level of evidence B)

Class III

1. Transient A-V block in the absence of intraventricular conduction defects (Level of evidence B)
2. Transient A-V block in the presence of isolated left anterior fascicular block (Level of evidence B)
3. Acquired left anterior fascicular block in the absence of A-V block (Level of evidence B)
4. Persistent first-degree A-V block in the presence of bundle-branch block that is old or age-indeterminate (Level of evidence B)

See Table 5-2 for definitions of classes and levels of evidence. (Adapted with permission from Gregoratos G, Abrams J, Epstein AE, et al. ACC/AHA/NASPE 2002 guideline update for implantation of cardiac pacemakers and antiarrhythmia devices—summary article. *J Am Coll Cardiol.* 2002;40:1703–1719. Copyright 2002 by the American College of Cardiology and American Heart Association, Inc.[13])

LANDMARK CLINICAL TRIALS

See Table 5-5.

TABLE 5-5 Pacemaker placement

Intervention	Trial	Details
Dual chamber pacing vs. medical management for vasovagal syncope	VPS (*J Am Coll Cardiol* 1999[14]) N = 54	Dual chamber pacing with rate-drop response → 85.4% RRR in first recurrence of syncope. NNT = 2
Pacing with rate drop sensing vs. sensing alone and the risk of vasovagal syncope	VPS II (*Card Electrophysiol Rev* 2003[15]) N = 100	Pacing with rate drop sensing → 23% RRR in risk of syncope at 6 mo. NNT = 11
Atrial vs. ventricular pacing in sick-sinus syndrome	Prospective randomized trial of atrial vs. ventricular pacing in sick-sinus syndrome (*Lancet* 1994[16]) N = 225	Atrial pacing → 69% RRR of thromboembolic events at 5 y. NNT = 8

REFERENCES

1. Ufberg JW, Clark, JS. Bradydysrhythmias and atrioventricular conduction blocks. *Emerg Med Clin North Am.* 2006;24:1–9.
2. Olgin JE, Zipes DP. Specific arrhythmias: Diagnosis and treatment. In: Braunwald E, Zipes DP, Libby P, eds. *Braunwald's Heart Disease: A Textbook of Cardiovascular Medicine.* 6th ed. Philadelphia: WB Saunders; 2001:815–889.
3. Sandoe E, Sigurd B. *Arrhythmia—a Guide to Clinical Electrocardiology.* Verlags GmbH: Bingen Publishing Partners; 1991:278–290.
4. Shaw DB, Southall DP. Sinus node arrest and sino-atrial block. *Eur Heart J.* 1984;5(Suppl A):83–87.
5. Suawicz B, Knilans TK. *Chou's Electrocardiography in Clinical Practice.* 5th ed. Philadelphia: WB Saunders; 2001:321.
6. AnaesthesiaUK. ECG Interpretation: Conduction Abnormalities, 2006. http://www.frca.co.uk/article.aspx?articleid=100685
7. Rardon DP, Miles WM, Zipes DP. Atrioventricular block and dissociation. In: Zipes DP, Jalife J, eds. *Cardiac Electrophysiology: From Cell to Bedside.* 3rd ed. Philadelphia: WB Saunders; 2000:451–459.
8. Denes P, Levy L, Pick A, et al. The incidence of typical and atypical A-V Wenckebach periodicity. *Am Heart J.* 1975;89:26–31.
9. Bradycardia. ClinicalResource@Ovid Clin-eguide.
10. Hongo RH, Goldschlager NF. Bradycardia and pacemakers. In Wachter RM, Goldman L, Hollander H, eds. *Hospital Medicine.* 2nd ed. Philadelphia: Lippincott Williams & Wilkins. 2005.

11. Benditt DG, Benson DW Jr, Kreitt J, et al. Electrophysiologic effects of theophylline in young patients with recurrent symptomatic bradyar-rhythmias. *Am J Cardiol.*1983 Dec 1;52(10):1223–1229.

12. 2005 American Heart Association Guidelines for Cardiopulmonary Resuscitation and Emergency Cardiovascular Care; Part 7.3: Man-agement of Symptomatic Bradycardia and Tachycardia. *Circulation.* 2005;112:IV-67–IV-77.

13. Gregoratos G, Abrams J, Epstein AE, et al. ACC/AHA/NASPE 2002 guideline update for implantation of cardiac pace-makers and antiarrhythmia devices—summary article. *J Am Coll Cardiol.* 2002;40:1703–1719.

14. Connolly SJ, Sheldon R, Roberts RS, et al. The North American Vaso-vagal Pacemaker Study (VPS). A randomized trial of permanent cardiac pacing for the prevention of vasovagal syncope. *J Am Coll Cardiol.* 1999 Jan;33(1):16–20.

15. Sheldon R, Connolly S, Vasovagal Pacemaker Study II Investigators. Second Vasovagal Pacemaker Study (VPS II): Rationale, design, results, and implications for practice and future clinical trials *Card Electrophysiol Rev.* 2003 Dec;7(4):411–415.

16. Andersen HR, Thuesen L, Bagger JP, et al. Prospective randomized trial of atrial versus ventricular pacing in sick-sinus syndrome. *Lancet.* 1994 Dec 3;344(8936):1523–1528.

CHAPTER 6

Wide and Narrow Complex Tachyarrhythmias

DAVID V. DANIELS AND AMIN AL-AHMAD

BACKGROUND AND APPROACH

The tachyarrhythmias presented in this chapter and the approach to their differential diagnosis, workup, and treatment are among the most common problems encountered in inpatient cardiology. These entities range in gravity from arrhythmias that are a nuisance, allowing for careful consideration as to the best approach, to life-threatening emergencies demanding decisive action.

DEFINITIONS

- Narrow complex tachycardia: QRS duration <120 milliseconds
- Wide complex tachycardia: QRS duration >120 milliseconds with or without pre-excitation
- Pre-excitation: Initial "slurring" of the QRS complex implying manifest antegrade conduction down an accessory bypass tract (e.g., WPW pattern); may see in sinus rhythm atrial fibrillation (AF), or antidromic reciprocating tachycardia (ART)
- Supraventricular tachycardia (SVT): A tachycardia arising from or involving the atria, specialized atrial conduction tissue, or compact A-V node
- Though technically SVT includes AF, some exclude AF as a separate entity for the purposes of nomenclature for multiple reasons

* Ventricular tachycardia (VT): A tachycardia arising from and exclusively involving the tissue beneath the compact portion of the A-V node, including the His bundle, bundle branches, and ventricular myocardium
* VT most commonly associated with CAD and/or structural heart disease
* 10% of VT occurs in structurally normal hearts arising both from the endocardium[1,2] and epicardium[3]

HISTORY

* Symptoms include palpitations, dyspnea, chest pain, presyncope, syncope
* History of myocardial infraction (MI), congestive heart failure (CHF) increase the risk of malignant arrhythmias such as VT
* Implantable cardioverter-defibrillator (ICD) → consider VT
* Drop attack (sudden syncope without prodrome) is suggestive of cardiac mediated syncope but its absence should not dissuade you from considering the diagnosis[4]
* Palpitations are also commonly felt in the recovery phase of neurocardiogenic syncope
* Consider the patient's medications as an etiology of arrhythmias:

  ○ A-V nodal agents—see bradyarrhythmias
  ○ Antiarrhythmics—particularly those that prolong the QTc, IC agents (Flecainide, encainide (not available in the United States), propafenone), dofetilide, sotalol, amiodarone
  ○ QTc-prolonging nonantiarrhythmics—macrolides, fluoroquinolones, antipsychotics, etc.
  ○ Digoxin toxicity

PHYSICAL EXAM

* Hypotension or clinical instability does *not* distinguish between SVT and VT!
* Cannon A waves may be observed in the jugular venous pulse and in the setting of a wide complex tachycardia are indicative of A-V dissociation and highly suggestive of ventricular tachycardia
* Crackles or wheezes may suggest heart failure but also consider concomitant pulmonary disease that may be associated with atrial tachycardias
* Examine chest wall for the presence of an ICD or pacemaker that you can interrogate to reveal the atrial rhythm in difficult cases
* Murmurs may point to cardiac disease in general, which is useful, but an S3 is suggestive of decompensated heart failure and can be the cause or result of an arrhythmia

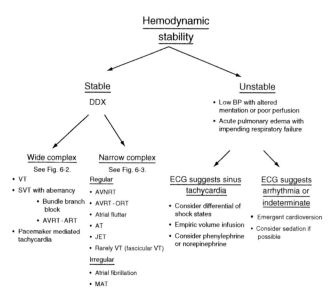

FIGURE 6-1 Algorithm for initial approach to tachyarrhythmias. DDX, differential diagnosis; VT, ventricular tachycardia; SVT, supraventricular tachycardia; AVRT, atrioventricular reentrant tachycardia; ART, antidromic reciprocating tachycardia; ORT, orthodromic reciprocating tachycardia; AVNRT, A-V nodal reentrant tachycardia; AT, atrial tachycardia; JET, junctional ectopic tachycardia.

INITIAL MANAGEMENT

* *Always consider cardioversion for unstable arrhythmias.* (See Figure 6-1.)
* Obtain a baseline ECG for comparison whenever possible!
* Attention to electrolyte abnormalities, especially ↓ K^+ and Mg^{2+}
* If the patient has an ICD or pacemaker (particularly dual chamber), consider interrogation to help with workup of the arrhythmia

WIDE COMPLEX TACHYCARDIA (WCT)

* Differential diagnosis includes VT versus SVT with aberrancy or pre-excited tachycardias. (See Table 6-1.)
  * Unselected population 80% of WCT = VT
  * Post-MI or structural heart disease 95% of WCT = VT[5]

- ○ Consider AF with antegrade conduction down an accessory pathway (pre-excited AF) if irregular with wide complex—avoid A-V nodal blockers can → VF
- ● Misdiagnosis of a WCT as SVT when it is VT can have several consequences:
  - ○ Acute progressive pump failure possible with incessant VT
  - ○ Drugs: Verapamil, diltiazem, adenosine are potentially dangerous in VT
  - ○ Failure to consider acute ischemia as an etiology of new onset VT

TABLE 6-1	Wide complex tachycardia: Differentiating VT from SVT	
Diagnostic Features	Ventricular Tachycardia	SVT with Aberrancy
Prior MI or structural heart disease	More likely	Less likely
WCT different in morphology from baseline QRS widening	More likely	Less likely
Right superior QRS axis	More likely	Less likely
A-V dissociation	Diagnostic	
Fusion or capture beats	Diagnostic	
Negative or positive concordance	>90% specific[6]	
V1 positive WCT (RBBB pattern)[7]	V1: rsR' (second R wave taller) >50:1 LR for VT V6: rS (small r, large S) >50:1 LR for VT	
V1 negative WCT (LBBB pattern)[7]	V1: Broad initial R wave >40 ms favors VT	Absence of an R wave or <40 ms favors SVT
	V1: Nadir of S wave >60 ms after initiation of QRS	Nadir of S wave <60 ms after initiation of QRS
	V6: Q or QS favors VT LR >50:1	Absence of Q wave favors SVT

Therefore, approach WCT with a prejudice toward the diagnosis of VT and consider SVT w/ aberrancy less likely unless supported by strong evidence.

Approach to Wide Complex Tachycardias:
Specific VT syndromes
* Polymorphic VT with normal QT interval: Strongly consider acute ischemia as the etiology
* Torsade de pointes

  ○ Polymorphic VT in the presence of a prolonged QT
  ○ Etiologies: drugs (www.torsades.org), ischemia, familial

* Idiopathic VT: VT in the absence of structural heart disease

  ○ RVOT VT, ILVT, LVOT VT, epicardial VT, aortic cusp VT

* Arrhythmogenic right ventricular dysplasia (ARVD): Epsilon wave
* Brugada syndrome: Characteristic atypical RBBB with ST elevation (leads to VF rather than VT)
* Bidirectional VT: Associated with digoxin toxicity

NARROW COMPLEX TACHYCARDIA

Every EKG has a differential diagnosis and the various mechanisms below should be listed as a definitive diagnosis which is usually difficult by EKG.

* Almost always SVT
* AVNRT is the most common cause of paroxysmal SVT in adults (50%), followed by AVRT (40%) and AT/SNRT (10%)[8]
* If irregular, likely AF or multifocal atrial tachycardia (MAT)
* If regular, rhythm useful to divide into short R-P, long R-P, or no R-P where the "R-P" interval is defined as the onset of the R wave → P wave

  ○ Short R-P tachycardia: R-P interval < P-R interval: AVNRT, AVRT, atypical atrial tachycardia (AT)
  ○ Long R-P tachycardia: R-P interval > P-R interval: Sinus tachycardia, SNRT, AT, atypical AVRT and AVNRT
  ○ No R-P tachycardia (no visible P waves): AVNRT most likely, atrial flutter, rarely AT or JET

* Rarely fascicular VT can present with minimally prolonged QRS, also can terminate with verapamil or diltiazem and therefore mimic SVT[9]

Approach to Narrow Complex Tachycardias:
Notes on Valsalva and Carotid Massage
* In an unselected population Valsalva followed by carotid sinus massage terminated PSVT in 28% of patients[10]

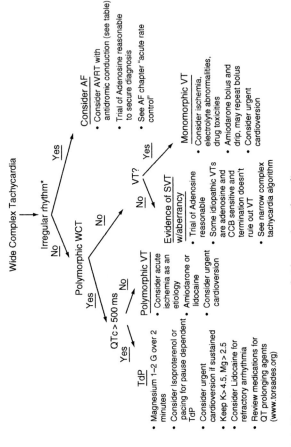

FIGURE 6-2 Algorithm for the management of wide complex tachycardias.

* VT can occasionally be irregular especially during initiation

= If WCT is actually VT, adenosine can precipitate VF, have defibrillation immediately available

Wide Complex Tachycardia

Irregular rhythm*

Yes

Consider AF
• Consider AVRT with antidromic conduction (see table)
• Trial of Adenosine reasonable to secure diagnosis
• See AF chapter "acute rate control"

No

QTc > 500 ms

Yes

TdP
• Magnesium 1-2 G over 2 minutes
• Consider Isoproterenol or pacing for pause dependent TdP
• Consider urgent cardioversion if sustained
• Keep K> 4.5, Mg > 2.5
• Consider Lidocaine for refractory arrhythmia
• Review medications for QT prolonging agents (www.torsades.org)

No

Polymorphic WCT

Yes

Polymorphic VT
• Consider acute ischemia as an etiology
• Amiodarone or lidocaine
• Consider urgent cardioversion

No

VT?

No

Evidence of SVT w/aberrancy
• Trial of Adenosine reasonable
• Some idiopathic VTs are adenosine and CCB sensitive and termination doesn't rule out VT
• See narrow complex tachycardia algorithm

Yes

Monomorphic VT
• Consider ischemia, electrolyte abnormalities, drug toxicities
• Amiodarone bolus and drip, may repeat bolus
• Consider urgent cardioversion

• In the absence of carotid bruits, history of stroke, MI within 6 months, history of VT or VF 11 neurologic complications in 16,000 occurrences of carotid sinus massage (CSM) and only 2 had permanent disability[11]

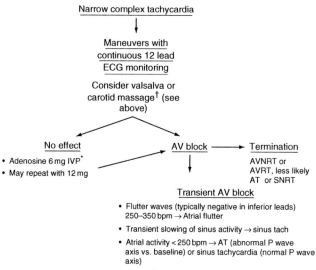

FIGURE 6-3 Algorithm for the management of narrow complex tachycardias. A-V block, atrioventricular block; AT, atrial tachycardia; AVNRT, atrioventricular nodal reentrant tachycardia; AVRT, atrioventricular reentrant tachycardia; JET, junctional ectopic tachycardia; SNRT, sinus node reentrant tachycardia

* Caution with WPW pattern on baseline ECG, can→ AF → VF (have defibrillator immediately available)

† Contraindicated with carotid bruits, history of stroke, MI within 6 months, history of VT or VF

PHARMACOLOGIC THERAPY OF TACHYARRHYTHMIAS

See Table 6-2.

TABLE 6-2	Pharmacologic therapy of tachyarrhythmias		
Arrhythmia	Drug	Dose	Notable side effects
VT	**Amiodarone**	150 mg IV over 10 min, then 1 mg/min infusion, consider reduction to 0.5 mg/min when stable or the patient develops sinus node supression	↓BP (though less significant than CCB and βB), HB, ↓HR, ventricular arrhythmia (attention to QTc), phlebitis with prolonged peripheral infusion, pulmonary toxicity, hepatotoxicity, hyper- or hypothyroidism, ocular toxicity, skin discoloration, warfarin and digoxin interaction
	Lidocaine	1–1.5 mg/kg IVP, may repeat in 5–10 min up to max 3 mg/kg	Tremor, insomnia, drowsiness, dysarthria, ataxia, seizures
		1–4 mg/min infusion Therapeutic level: 1.5–5.0 μg/mL	Sinus slowing, asystole Nausea, vomiting
	Procainamide	15–18 mg/kg over 30 min, then 1-4 mg/min	↓BP, torsade de pointes, nausea, vomiting, diarrhea
		Renal impairment (RI) reduce load to 12 mg/kg and infusion 1/3 mild and 2/3 severe RI	Cross allergy Avoid with QTc >500 ms
Torsade de pointes	**Magnesium**	1–2 g over 10 min	
	Lidocaine	As above	
	Isoproterenol Consider for TdP associated with significant bradycardia	2 μg/min (range 2–10 μg/min)	PVCs, VT, tachycardia, worsening of ischemia, tremor (the "Isuprel shakes"), nausea, vomiting, hypokalemia, hyperglycemia
SVT *without* pre-excitation	**Adenosine**	6 mg IVP, repeat with 12 mg if no A-V block Give rapidly via proximal peripheral IV with rapid flush Central line preferred if already in place	↓BP, asystole, AF, facial flushing (up to 45%, warn patients of this!), bronchospasm, chest pain, dyspnea

Arrhythmia	Drug	Dose	Notable side effects
	Esmolol	0.5 mg/kg IV over 1 min; may repeat q 4 min while titrating *infusion*: 50–200 µg/kg/min	↓BP, HB, ↓HR, bronchospasm, HF; exercise extreme caution if used despite HF or hypotension though very short half-life
	Metoprolol	2.5 to 5 mg IV over 2 min; may repeat q 5 min up to 3 doses	↓BP, HB, ↓HR, bronchospasm, HF; exercise extreme caution if used despite HF or hypotension
	Diltiazem	0.25 mg/kg (~20 mg) IV over 2 min; may repeat in 15 min at dose of 0.35 mg/kg (~25 mg) IV over 2 min *infusion*: 5–15 mg/h	↓BP, HB, HF; exercise extreme caution if used despite HF or hypotension
	Verapamil	0.075 to 0.15 mg/kg (~5–10 mg) IV over 2 min; may repeat in 15–30 min *infusion*: 0.125 mg/min	↓BP, HB, HF; contraindicated in HF or hypotension
SVT with pre-excitation	**Procainamide**	As above	As above
	Amiodarone	As above, not FDA approved but reasonable	As above
SVT with heart failure	**Amiodarone**	As above, not FDA approved but reasonable	As above
AF	See chapter on AF		

Modified from Fuster V, Ryden LE, Cannom DS, et al. ACC/AHA/ESC 2006 Guidelines for the Management of Patients with Atrial Fibrillation: A report of the American College of Cardiology/American Heart Association Task Force on Practice Guidelines and the European Society of Cardiology Committee for Practice Guidelines (Writing Committee to Revise the 2001 Guidelines for the Management of Patients With Atrial Fibrillation): Developed in collaboration with the European Heart Rhythm Association and the Heart Rhythm Society. *Circulation.* 2006;114(7):e257–354.[12]

REFERENCES

1. Wilber DJ, Baerman J, Olshansky B, et al. Adenosine-sensitive ventricular tachycardia. Clinical characteristics and response to catheter ablation. *Circulation.* 1993;87(1):126–134.

2. Ohe T, Shimomura K, Aihara N, et al. Idiopathic sustained left ventricular tachycardia: Clinical and electrophysiologic characteristics. *Circulation.* 1988;77(3):560–568.

3. Daniels DV, Lu YY, Morton JB, et al. Idiopathic epicardial left ventricular tachycardia originating remote from the sinus of Valsalva: Electrophysiological characteristics, catheter ablation, and identification from the 12-lead electrocardiogram. *Circulation.* 2006;113(13): 1659–1666.

4. Fuster V, Alexander RW, O'Rourke RA. *Hurst's the Heart.* 11th ed. New York: McGraw-Hill Medical Publishing Division; 2004.

5. Tchou P, Young P, Mahmud R, et al. Useful clinical criteria for the diagnosis of ventricular tachycardia. *Am J Med.* 1988;84(1):53–56.

6. Zipes DP, Jalife J. *Cardiac Electrophysiology: From Cell to Bedside.* 4th ed. Philadelphia: WB Saunders; 2004.

7. Lau EW, Pathamanathan RK, Ng GA, et al. The Bayesian approach improves the electrocardiographic diagnosis of broad complex tachycardia. *Pacing Clin Electrophysiol.* 2000;23(10 Pt 1):1519–1526.

8. Josephson ME. *Clinical Cardiac Electrophysiology: Techniques and Interpretations.* 3rd ed. Philadelphia: Lippincott Williams & Wilkins; 2002.

9. Elswick BD, Niemann JT. Fascicular ventricular tachycardia: An uncommon but distinctive form of ventricular tachycardia. *Ann Emerg Med.* 1998;31(3):406–409.

10. Lim SH, Anantharaman V, Teo WS, et al. Comparison of treatment of supraventricular tachycardia by Valsalva maneuver and carotid sinus massage. *Ann Emerg Med.* 1998;31(1):30–35.

11. Davies AJ, Kenny RA. Frequency of neurologic complications following carotid sinus massage. *Am J Cardiol.* 1998;81(10):1256–1257.

12. Fuster V, Ryden LE, Cannom DS, et al. ACC/AHA/ESC 2006 Guidelines for the Management of Patients with Atrial Fibrillation: A report of the American College of Cardiology/American Heart Association Task Force on Practice Guidelines and the European Society of Cardiology Committee for Practice Guidelines (Writing Committee to Revise the 2001 Guidelines for the Management of Patients With Atrial Fibrillation): Developed in collaboration with the European Heart Rhythm Association and the Heart Rhythm Society. *Circulation.* 2006;114(7):e257–354.

CHAPTER 7

Sudden Cardiac Death and ICD Therapy

DAVID V. DANIELS AND HENRY HSIA

BACKGROUND

Sudden cardiac death (SCD) is defined as death from cardiovascular causes shortly after the onset of symptoms in a person without a condition that would otherwise appear fatal.[1] Estimates as to the impact of SCD on our health care system put the total annual mortality up to 450,000, which is 63% of all deaths from cardiovascular causes.[2] Mechanisms of arrhythmic SCD include[3,4]:

- Ventricular arrhythmia (60% to 80%): Most commonly VT → VF, also primary VF, or torsade de pointes
- Bradyarrhythmia/asystole
- Pulseless electrical activity (PEA)

In a series of young sudden death patients <40 years old without known heart disease, the most common etiology was still cardiac (73%). Coronary heart disease (CHD) was the most common cause in those >30 (58%), while myocarditis (22%), hypertrophic cardiomyopathy (HCM) (22%), and conduction system disease (13%) were more common in those <20 years of age.[5] (See Table 7-1.)

TABLE 7-1	Etiologies of sudden death	
Structural (up to 75%)	**Primary electrical (5%–10%)**	**Noncardiac (10%–35%)**
• Coronary heart disease • Dilated cardiomyopathy • Hypertrophic obstructive cardiomyopathy (HOCM) • Coronary anomalies • Valvular disease • Hypertensive heart disease and LVH • Arrhythmogenic right ventricular dysplasia (ARVD) • Inflammatory and infiltrative myocardial disease • Ventricular noncompaction • Congenital heart disease	• Congenital or acquired long QT syndrome • Idiopathic polymorphic VT and VF • Brugada syndrome • WPW • Proarrhythmia associated with drugs • Toxic/metabolic • Commotio cordis • Short QT syndrome	• Intracranial hemorrhage (most common) • Pulmonary embolism • Trauma • Bleeding • Drug intoxication • Near drowning • Central airway obstruction

OUTCOMES

SCD is associated with a high incidence of mortality, and the ability to rescue the patient probably depends most on timely interventions that restore perfusion to and protect vital organs. Unfortunately, many patients will die in the prehospital setting or early in the resuscitative effort. For out-of-hospital sudden death, 20% make it to the hospital, half of them will die in the hospital, and only about half of the survivors will have any "meaningful" survival. Hence in total only about 5% of patients who sustain an out-of-hospital sudden death in the absence of ICD therapy will have a good outcome. In contrast, the survival with early defibrillation when the initial rhythm is VT or VF is substantially higher with up to 40% of those being discharged with a good neurologic outcome and is the single factor most strongly associated with a good outcome.[4,6] Those that regain a sustained perfusing rhythm are candidates for further therapy as outlined in Figure 7-1.

INITIAL PREDICTORS OF POOR PROGNOSIS

• Prolonged resuscitation time (>20 minutes)
• Survival decreases by ~10% for each minute of lapsed time before restoration of a viable rhythm

- Asystole (0% to 2% survival) or pulseless electrical activity (PEA) (11% survival) as the initial rhythm
- End tidal CO_2 by capnography <10 mm Hg after 20 minutes of resuscitation in patients with PEA predicts death with 100% sensitivity and specificity[7]

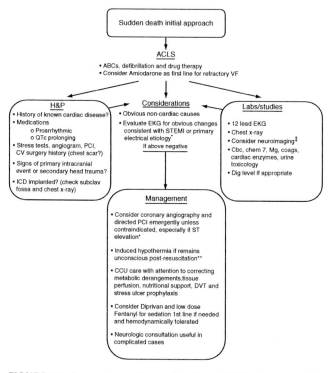

FIGURE 7-1 Approach to sudden cardiac death. ACLS, advanced cardiac life support; ABC, airway, breathing, circulation; VF, ventricular fibrillation; PCI, percutaneous coronary intervention; ICD, internal cardioverter defibrillator; CCU, coronary care unit; DVT, deep venous thrombosis
* See above for details.
‡ Especially if planned angiography. Intracranial hemorrhage is the most common noncardiac cause of sudden death. Also trauma secondary to cardiac arrest may → bleeding which can be complicated by therapeutic anticoagulation.
** See following for details.

SPECIFIC ACUTE THERAPIES

Coronary Angiography and Directed Revascularization[8]
- High degree of obstructive coronary artery disease (CAD) (71%) in an unselected population of SCD
- Up to 50% have a totally occluded coronary artery
- ST elevation + chest pain are highly predictive of recent coronary occlusion (87%), ST elevation alone (63%)
- Up to 25% of those with recent total coronary occlusions have *NO* pathologic ST elevation
- Successful angioplasty is an independent predictor of survival (Odds ratio 5.2)
- Therefore, coronary angiography is reasonable in all survivors of SCD, especially in those with persistent ST elevation or antecedent chest pain, but should be considered on an individual basis for all patients given the significant pretest probability of obstructive CAD and potential for decreasing further arrhythmic events

Induced Hypothermia Protocol
- Consider for patients who do not regain consciousness immediately after cardiac arrest
- Well validated in combination with primary PCI after resuscitation[9]
- Induced hypothermia 32-34 degrees Celsius by cooling blankets, ice packs, or central venous cooling catheter for 24 hours followed by passive rewarming[10,11]
- Monitor temperature with bladder or central venous temperature probe
- Sedation with midazolam or Diprivan, analgesia with fentanyl, paralysis with nondepolarizing neuromuscular blocking agent to prevent shivering
- Bradycardia is common during hypothermia but seldom requires treatment[11]

Further Testing
In the absence of CHD, other less common structural, metabolic, and primary electrical etiologies should be considered. The following provide a framework for this investigation:

Review of History
- History of known structural heart disease: prior myocardial infarct/ coronary artery disease (MI/CAD), hypertrophic cardiomyopathy (HCM), rheumatic heart disease, valvular CM, dilated cardiomyopathy (DCM)
- Family history: FH of SCD, LQT syndrome, FH of CAD, WPW, etc.
- Medication list: drugs known to cause long QT

Evaluation of the 12-Lead ECG for Primary Electrical Etiologies of SCD

- Look for evidence of structural heart disease:
  - Q waves for transmural scar from prior MI
  - Evidence of LVH, sarcoidosis (blocks)
  - Amyloidosis (low volts), epsilon wave for arrhythmogenic right ventricular dysplasia (ARVD)
  - Consider congenital or acquired long QT syndrome in a patient with significantly prolonged QTc, risk of torsade is low with a QTc <500 milliseconds[12]

- Pre-excitation suggestive of a bypass tract which could → rapid A-V conduction and VF
- Brugada syndrome:
  - Atypical ST elevation in V1-V3, right bundle branch block pattern[13]
  - Associated with polymorphic VT and VF

- Congenital short QT syndrome:
  - Very rare, manifest by QTc <300 milliseconds[14]

Echocardiography

- Looks for anatomical correlates of the underlying substrate: Wall motion abnormalities, aneurysm for scar-based arrhythmic substrate (Table 7-1)
- May reveal evidence of left ventricular hypertrophy (LVH), dilated cardiomyopathy (DCM), HCM, significant valvular disease, pulmonary hypertension, acute RV failure suggestive of possible pulmonary embolism
- While often performed early, should consider repeating if abnormal LV function >48 hours after resuscitation because early myocardial stunning may improve[11]

Cardiac MRI

- Useful for evaluation of myocarditis, ARVD, infiltrative cardiomyopathies, and occult myocardial infarction and scar
- Correlates with increased progression of disease and risk factors for sudden death in patients with hypertrophic cardiomyopathy (HCM)[15]
- Late gadolinium enhancement correlates with risk of SCD in patients with nonischemic cardiomyopathy[16]
- Contraindicated with pacemakers, ICD, or ferromagnetic medical devices

Electrophysiology Study

- Primarily indicated in those with an accessory pathway (WPW pattern) to assess the anterograde properties of the accessory pathways,

shortest RR during pre-excited AF, ERP of the pathway, followed by RFA
* Recurrent refractory ventricular arrhythmias, myocardial scar
* In pts who had a SCD and sustained monomorphic VT is suspected, in a setting of MI, to induce VT and determine the number, morphology, rate of VT and its response to antitachycardia pacing (ATP) → for future ICD programming
* Except in the case of a clear link to an accessory pathway → sudden death, most patients should still get an ICD despite RF ablation

SECONDARY PREVENTION

ICD Therapy
* Significant mortality benefit in survivors of SCD when compared to amiodarone[17]
* Likely greater benefit in those with left ventricular ejection fraction (LVEF) <35%[17]
* Careful consideration of contraindications including:

  ○ Noncardiac disease associated with high short-term mortality
  ○ Active proarrhythmic illegal drug use

Beta Blockers
* Beta blockade is associated with significant reductions in mortality in systolic heart failure from both reductions in progressive pump failure and sudden death.[18,19]

Amiodarone
* In contrast to most other antiarrhythmic drugs (see Table 7-2), amiodarone is not pro-arrhythmic and *not* associated with increased mortality[20]
* Meta-analysis confirms no statistically significant mortality benefit in post-MI, LV dysfunction and postcardiac arrest versus placebo[21]
* Should *not* replace beta blockers if indicated for heart failure as they have proven mortality benefit and careful combination therapy is generally safe[22]
* Should *not* replace ICD therapy but may consider as an adjunct to reduce shocks
* Toxicities and intolerance → discontinuation or dose reduction in up to 50% long term[23]
* 800 to 1200 mg/day in divided doses while in hospital, 400 mg/day for 3 to 4 weeks, 200 mg/day maintenance
* Attention to toxicities: Baseline and interval TSH, PFTs (w/ DLCO), chest X-ray, LFTs, Optho exam

Antiarrhythmic therapy of aborted sudden cardiac death

Arrhythmia	Drug	Dose	Notable acute side effects
Monomorphic VT or VF	**Amiodarone**	If pulseless 300 mg IVP, then 1 mg/min If cardioverted and stable, 150 mg IV over 10 min, then 1 mg/min, consider reduction to 0.5 mg/min when stable	Relatively contraindicated with congenital or acquired long QT syndrome ↓BP (though less significant than CCB and βB), HB, ↓HR, ventricular arrhythmia (attention to QTc), phlebitis with prolonged peripheral infusion
	Lidocaine	1–1.5 mg/kg IVP, may repeat 0.5/0.75 mg/kg in 5–10 min up to max 3 mg/kg 1–4 mg/min infusion Therapeutic level: 1.5–5.0 µg/mL	Tremor, insomnia, drowsiness, dysarthria, ataxia, seizures Sinus slowing, asystole Nausea, vomiting
	Procainamide	15–18 mg/kg over 30 min, then 1–4 mg/min Renal impairment (RI) reduce load to 12 mg/kg and infusion 1/3 mild and 2/3 severe RI	↓BP, torsade de pointes, nausea, vomiting, diarrhea Cross allergy with ester-type local anasthetics Avoid with QTc >500 ms
Torsade de pointes (TdP)	**Magnesium**	1–2 g IV over 10 min	
	Isoproterenol Consider for TdP associated with significant bradycardia	2 µg/min (range 2–10 µg/min)	PVCs, VT, tachycardia, worsening of ischemia, tremor, nausea, vomiting, hypokalemia, hypoglycemia
	Transvenous pacing	HR 80–100, especially useful for TdP associated with bradycardia	

LANDMARK CLINICAL TRIALS

See Table 7-3.

TABLE 7-3	Landmark clinical trials	
Intervention	Trial	Details
Acute therapies		
Coronary angiography with directed PCI	Spaulding et al. (N Engl J Med 1997[8]) n = 84	Odds ratio 5.2 (95% CI 1.2–24.5) for survival in patients with successful angioplasty
Induced moderate hypothermia (H) in postarrest patients with persistent coma vs. normothermia (N)	Bernard et al. (N Engl J Med 2002[11]) n = 77	Hypothermia → 53% RRR (N 49% H 26%) of bad neurologic outcome **NNT = 5**
Combined PCI and induced hypothermia (H) in survivors of cardiac arrest vs. normothermia (N)	Knafelj et al. (Resuscitation 2007[9]) n = 72	Hypothermia combined with PCI in patients with STEMI and cardiac arrest → 71% RRR (N 16% H 55%) of bad neurologic outcome **NNT = 3**
Antiarrhythmics		
Amiodarone vs. EPS guided antiarrhythmic therapy in survivors of SCD in the absence of AMI	CASCADE[24] (Am J Cardiol 1993) n = 228	Amiodarone → 50% RRR of death at 6 y vs. conventional therapy (most often type 1A antiarrhythmics which are associated with ↑ mortality) Avg. EF 35% **NNT = 5**
Amiodarone vs. placebo in post-MI patients with EF <40%	EMIAT[25] (Lancet 1997) n = 1,486	Amiodarone → 35% RRR of arrhythmic death (A 2.2%, P 3.3%) at 21 mo **NNT = 91** NO difference in mortality
Amiodarone vs. placebo in post-MI patients with frequent PVCs	CAMIAT[26] (Lancet 1997) n = 1,202	Amiodarone → 49% RRR of arrhythmic death (A 4.5%, P 6.9%) at 1.8 y **NNT = 42** NO difference in mortality

Amiodarone vs. placebo	Meta-analysis[21] *(Circulation 1997)* n = 5,864	Amiodarone → no statistically significant difference in all cause mortality

ICD Therapy

Secondary prevention

ICD vs. amiodarone in patients resuscitated from SCD or with hemodynamically significant VT	AVID[27] *(N Engl J Med 1997)* n = 1,016	ICD → 24% RRR of total mortality (A 24% I 15.8%) at 18 mo **NNT = 13**
ICD vs. amiodarone or metoprolol in survivors of SCD secondary to ventricular arrhythmias	CASH[28] *(Circulation 2000)* n = 288	ICD → 23% RRR of total mortality (A/M 44.4% I 36.4%, P 0.08) at 57 mo. P value not significant. N.b. procedural mortality was high (4%) early in the ICD group and trial was significantly underpowered
ICD vs. amiodarone	Meta-analysis (AVID/CASH/CIDS)[17] *(Eur Heart J)* n = 1,866	ICD → Hazard ratio 0.72 for total mortality (Annual mortality A 12.3% I 8.8%) ICD vs. amiodarone **NNT = 29**

Primary prevention

ICD vs. conventional therapy for primary prevention of SCD in post-MI with EF <30%	MADIT II[29] *(N Engl J Med 2002)* n = 1,232	ICD → 31% RRR of total mortality (C 19.8% I 14.2%) at 20 mo. Avg EF 23% **NNT = 18**
ICD vs. amiodarone vs. placebo with EF <35% and NYHA II or III CHF	SCD-HeFT[20] *(N Engl J Med 2005)* n = 2,521	ICD 23% RRR of total mortality (P 29% A 28% I 22%) at 4 y. Avg EF 25% No difference between amiodarone and placebo **NNT = 15**

REFERENCES

1. Goldstein S. The necessity of a uniform definition of sudden coronary death: Witnessed death within 1 hour of the onset of acute symptoms. *Am Heart J.* 1982;103(1):156–159.

2. Zheng ZJ, Croft JB, Giles WH, et al. Sudden cardiac death in the United States, 1989 to 1998. *Circulation.* 2001;104(18):2158–2163.

3. Bayes de Luna A, Coumel P, Leclercq JF. Ambulatory sudden cardiac death: Mechanisms of production of fatal arrhythmia on the basis of data from 157 cases. *Am Heart J.* 1989;117(1):151–159.

4. Rea TD, Eisenberg MS, Becker LJ, et al. Temporal trends in sudden cardiac arrest: A 25-year emergency medical services perspective. *Circulation.* 2003;107(22):2780–2785.

5. Drory Y, Turetz Y, Hiss Y, et al. Sudden unexpected death in persons less than 40 years of age. *Am J Cardiol.* 1991;68(13):1388–1392.

6. Bunch TJ, White RD, Gersh BJ, et al. Outcomes and in-hospital treatment of out-of-hospital cardiac arrest patients resuscitated from ventricular fibrillation by early defibrillation. *Mayo Clin Proc.* 2004;79(5):613–619.

7. Levine RL, Wayne MA, Miller CC. End-tidal carbon dioxide and outcome of out-of-hospital cardiac arrest. *N Engl J Med.* 1997; 337(5):301–306.

8. Spaulding CM, Joly LM, Rosenberg A, et al. Immediate coronary angiography in survivors of out-of-hospital cardiac arrest. *N Engl J Med.* 1997;336(23):1629–1633.

9. Knafelj A, Radsel A, Ploj A, et al. Primary percutaneous coronary intervention and mild induced hypothermia in comatose survivors of ventricular fibrillation with ST-elevation acute myocardial infarction. *Resuscitation.* 2007;74(2):227–234.

10. Al-Senani FM, Graffagnino C, Grotta JC, et al. A prospective, multicenter pilot study to evaluate the feasibility and safety of using the CoolGard System and Icy catheter following cardiac arrest. *Resuscitation.* 2004;62(2):143–150.

11. Bernard SA, Gray TW, Buist MD, et al. Treatment of comatose survivors of out-of-hospital cardiac arrest with induced hypothermia. *N Engl J Med.* 2002;346(8):557–563.

12. Bednar MM, Harrigan EP, Anziano RJ, et al. The QT interval. *Prog Cardiovasc Dis.* 2001;43(5 Suppl 1):1–45.

13. Antzelevitch C, Brugada P, Borggrefe M, et al. Brugada syndrome: Report of the second consensus conference: Endorsed by the Heart Rhythm Society and the European Heart Rhythm Association. *Circulation.* 2005;111(5):659–670.

14. Gaita F, Giustetto C, Bianchi F, et al. Short QT Syndrome: A familial cause of sudden death. *Circulation.* 2003;108(8): 965–970.

15. Moon JCC, McKenna WJ, McCrohon JA, et al. Toward clinical risk assessment in hypertrophic cardiomyopathy with gadolinium cardiovascular magnetic resonance. *J Am Coll Cardiol.* 2003;41(9):1561–1567.

16. Assomull RG, Prasad SK, Lyne J, et al. Cardiovascular magnetic resonance, fibrosis, and prognosis in dilated cardiomyopathy. *J Am Coll Cardiol.* 2006;48(10):1977–1985.

17. Connolly SJ, Hallstrom AP, Cappato R, et al. Meta-analysis of the implantable cardioverter defibrillator secondary prevention trials. AVID, CASH and CIDS studies. Antiarrhythmics vs Implantable Defibrillator study. Cardiac Arrest Study Hamburg. Canadian Implantable Defibrillator Study. *Eur Heart J.* 2000;21(24):2071–2078.

18. Goldstein S, Fagerberg B, Hjalmarson AJ, et al. Metoprolol controlled release/extended release in patients with severe heart failure: Analysis of the experience in the MERIT-HF study. *J Am Coll Cardiol.* 2001;38(4):932–938.

19. Packer M, Bristow MR, Cohn JN, et al. The effect of carvedilol on morbidity and mortality in patients with chronic heart failure. U.S. Carvedilol Heart Failure Study Group. *N Engl J Med.* 1996;334(21):1349–1355.

20. Bardy GH, Lee KL, Mark DB, et al. Amiodarone or an implantable cardioverter-defibrillator for congestive heart failure. *N Engl J Med.* 2005;352(3):225–237.

21. Sim I, McDonald KM, Lavori PW, et al. Quantitative overview of randomized trials of amiodarone to prevent sudden cardiac death. *Circulation.* 1997;96(9):2823–2829.

22. Bashir Y, Paul VE, Griffith MJ, et al. A prospective study of the efficacy and safety of adjuvant metoprolol and xamoterol in combination with amiodarone for resistant ventricular tachycardia associated with impaired left ventricular function. *Am Heart J.* 1992;124(5):1233–1240.

23. Bokhari F, Newman D, Greene M, et al. Long-term comparison of the implantable cardioverter defibrillator versus amiodarone: Eleven-year follow-up of a subset of patients in the Canadian Implantable Defibrillator Study (CIDS). *Circulation.* 2004;110(2):112–116.

24. Randomized antiarrhythmic drug therapy in survivors of cardiac arrest (the CASCADE Study). The CASCADE Investigators. *Am J Cardiol.* 1993;72(3):280–287.

25. Julian DG, Camm AJ, Frangin G, et al. Randomized trial of effect of amiodarone on mortality in patients with left-ventricular dysfunction after recent myocardial infarction: EMIAT. European Myocardial Infarct Amiodarone Trial Investigators. *Lancet.* 1997;349(9053):667–674.

26. Cairns JA, Connolly SJ, Roberts R, et al. Randomized trial of outcome after myocardial infarction in patients with frequent or repetitive ventricular premature depolarizations: CAMIAT. Canadian Amiodarone Myocardial Infarction Arrhythmia Trial Investigators. *Lancet.* 1997;349(9053):675–682.

27. A comparison of antiarrhythmic-drug therapy with implantable defibrillators in patients resuscitated from near-fatal ventricular arrhythmias. The Antiarrhythmics versus Implantable Defibrillators (AVID) Investigators. *N Engl J Med.* 1997;337(22):1576–1583.

28. Kuck KH, Cappato R, Siebels J, et al. Randomized comparison of antiarrhythmic drug therapy with implantable defibrillators in patients resuscitated from cardiac arrest: The Cardiac Arrest Study Hamburg (CASH). *Circulation.* 2000;102(7):748–754.
29. Moss AJ, Zareba W, Hall WJ, et al. Prophylactic implantation of a defibrillator in patients with myocardial infarction and reduced ejection fraction. *N Engl J Med.* 2002;346(12):877–883.

CHAPTER 8

Atrial Fibrillation

ANURAG GUPTA AND PAUL J. WANG

BACKGROUND

Atrial fibrillation (AF) is the most common chronic cardiac dysrhythmia. The estimated prevalence of atrial fibrillation and atrial flutter is greater than 2.2 million individuals in the United States, with estimated incidence of greater than 75,000 cases per year.[1] The median age of individuals with AF is approximately 75 years. The estimated lifetime risk for the development of AF, when studied in all individuals age 40 years or older free of AF in the Framingham Heart Study, was estimated to be approximately 1 in 4.[2] The morbidity and mortality attributable to AF is significant as its presence confers an increased risk for congestive heart failure (CHF), embolic events including stroke, and death.

ELECTROPHYSIOLOGIC FEATURES

AF is supraventricular arrhythmia characterized by seemingly disorganized atrial depolarizations consequently accompanied by ineffectual atrial contraction. The mechanisms contributing to AF are under investigation with proposed, possibly coexisting, models that include the following:

- *Multiple-wavelet reentry*, in which AF is maintained via multiple coexisting wave fronts of electrical activity that propagate randomly throughout the atria
- *Focal activation* at areas of enhanced automaticity, with rapid discharge leading to heterogeneous, fibrillatory conduction. Of note, numerous foci have been identified though the region of the pulmonary veins in the left atrium appears to be most common[3]
- *Small reentrant sources* (rotors) that lead to a hierarchical distribution of frequencies throughout the atria that maintain AF

- *Heterogeneity of autonomic innervation* likely plays a further role in the initiation and maintenance of AF

AF appears to be initiated by atrial premature beats (most commonly), as well as by atrial flutter and other supraventricular tachycardias.

ELECTROCARDIOGRAPHIC FEATURES[4]

The ECG appearance of AF is most immediately suggested by an irregular ventricular rhythm with no discrete P waves. More specifically,

- *Atrial activity*: P waves are replaced by f waves, typically smaller waves characterized by variable morphology, amplitude, and intervals, with rapid rate generally between 350 and 600 beats per minute (bpm).
- *Ventricular response*: The ventricular response (R-R interval) is generally irregular with rate of 90 to 170 bpm in an untreated individual. The ventricular rate is significantly less than the atrial rate due to block at the A-V node and possibly due to collision of fibrillatory wave fronts. However, the ventricular rate varies significantly depending upon multiple factors including
  - ○ action of drugs
  - ○ electrophysiological properties of the A-V node and conducting tissue
  - ○ autonomic tone
- *Accessory pathways?* Assess for the possible presence of an accessory pathway(s) capable of antegrade conduction, as ventricular rates can be greater than 300 bpm and deteriorate into lethal ventricular fibrillation. The presence of an accessory pathway may be suggested by typical appearance on an electrocardiogram during sinus rhythm (namely, short P-R interval with delta wave), by extremely rapid ventricular rates greater than 200 bpm during AF, and/or by wide-QRS complexes during AF (although aberrant conduction or pre-existing conduction abnormality can also lead to wide complexes).

INITIAL MANAGEMENT

1. Attempt to identify and address underlying etiologies, risk factors, and/or triggers for AF, including potentially reversible causes of AF
2. Initiate appropriate antithrombotic therapy, if indicated and safe, based on an individualized assessment of overall stroke risk
3. Control the ventricular rate, if needed
4. Assess the acute and/or chronic effects of AF including associated symptoms and its hemodynamic consequences. This will help guide decisions of whether or not to pursue a strategy of attempting to restore and maintain sinus rhythm.

CLINICAL CONSEQUENCES

Hemodynamic Compromise

The hemodynamic derangements in AF may or may not be accompanied with symptoms, most commonly palpitations, dyspnea, decreased exercise tolerance, lightheadedness, syncope, and chest discomfort. The factors leading to hemodynamic deterioration include the following:

* Loss of effective atrial contraction and thus atrioventricular (A-V) synchrony; this may be especially detrimental in those dependent upon diastolic ventricular filling
* Irregularity of ventricular response
* Inappropriately elevated heart rate. Chronically elevated atrial rates may lead to adverse atrial remodeling (including atrial dilatation), and persistently elevated ventricular rates may lead to the development of a tachycardia-induced cardiomyopathy. Excessive ventricular rates may also compromise diastolic ventricular filling.

Thromboembolic Risk

Multiple factors contribute to increased thromboembolic events in individuals with AF, although static flow within the left atrial appendage (LAA) appears most significant. The rate of ischemic stroke varies significantly depending upon the presence of associated stroke risk factors, but on average is estimated to be approximately 5% per year in individuals with nonvalvular AF (that is, AF not associated with rheumatic mitral valve disease, valve replacement, or valve repair). This represents an approximately six-fold increase in the risk of thromboembolic events in individuals with nonvalvular AF as compared to individuals without AF. The attributable risk of stroke in individuals with AF increases significantly with advancing age.[5]

CLASSIFICATION[6]

The following definitions apply to episodes of AF lasting longer than 30 seconds without a reversible cause. It is useful to identify a *first-detected episode* of AF, acknowledging that the duration of that episode is generally unknown and prior undetected episodes may have been present. When AF has been detected at least 2 times, it is termed *recurrent* AF.

First-detected or recurrent AF can be further classified as the following:

* *Paroxysmal*: AF episode(s) usually lasts 7 days or less (and most less than 24 hours) and terminates spontaneously
* *Persistent*: AF episode(s) usually lasts greater than 7 days and does not terminate spontaneously
* *Permanent*: Cardioversion has failed and/or attempts have been foregone

ETIOLOGIES

The delineation of the following risk factors for AF is somewhat arbitrary, overlap exists, and multiple etiologies are often present in one individual. Nonetheless, "secondary" AF is intended to draw attention to cases in which AF may not be the primary problem, and may be ameliorated or terminated by treatment of the underlying disorder.

"Primary" AF

Established risk factors for the development of AF include the following:

* Advancing age
* Hypertension (systemic and/or pulmonary), especially when accompanied by left ventricular hypertrophy
* Coronary heart disease, especially when complicated by history of myocardial infarction (MI) or CHF
* Valvular heart disease, especially mitral regurgitation, mitral stenosis, and tricuspid regurgitation. In developed nations, this etiology is decreasing in frequency due to the reduced incidence of rheumatic heart disease.
* Heart failure
* Other factors, possibly including hypertrophic cardiomyopathy, congenital heart disease, intracardiac (or adjacent) tumors or thrombi, obstructive sleep apnea, and obesity
* *Lone* or "idiopathic" AF is said to be present in individuals younger than 60 years of age with no known cardiopulmonary disease (including hypertension) per clinical and echocardiographic assessment. The risk profile, including thromboembolic complications and death, is typically lower, though these individuals generally progress beyond the lone AF category with time. Multiple factors including genetic determinants, "sick sinus" syndrome, degenerative conduction disease, and other electrophysiologic abnormalities likely account for a significant proportion of incident AF but their role remains incompletely defined at present.

"Secondary" AF

Potentially reversible, "acute" *causes and/or triggers* for AF include the following:

* Acute MI (usually as a complication of transmural ST segment elevation MI [STEMI])
* Pericarditis
* Myocarditis
* Endocrine disorders including uncontrolled hyperthyroidism and pheochromocytoma
* Infection
* Postoperative state, especially with cardiac, pulmonary, or esophageal interventions

- Acute pulmonary disease, such as pulmonary embolus, pneumonia, and exacerbation of obstructive lung disease
- Neurogenic disease, such as major stroke and subarachnoid hemorrhage
- Toxins, such as alcohol, cocaine, amphetamines, and caffeine, including withdrawal states
- Medications, such as theophylline or positive inotropes
- Electrolyte disturbance, such as hypokalemia and hypomagnesemia
- Other supraventricular arrhythmias
- Enhanced sympathetic or parasympathetic tone

EVALUATION

It is critical to carefully consider in every single patient potential etiologies and risk factors predisposing one to AF. This provides an opportunity to identify and modify significant concomitant medical disease. However, one must be cognizant that even despite correction of a suspected reversible cause of AF, a patient may have underlying paroxysmal AF necessitating long-term therapy.

To evaluate possible etiologies of AF and to guide management decisions, it is reasonable to obtain the following diagnostics, with further studies guided by the clinical scenario.

History and Physical Examination

Characterize the patient's pattern of AF; define her symptoms; document her response to prior therapies; identify possible etiologies, risk factors, and triggers; and assess for clinical evidence of heart failure.

ECG

Verify the presence of AF, assess for accessory pathways, determine ventricular rate, document concomitant cardiac disease (e.g., atrial size, left ventricular hypertrophy [LVH], prior MI), monitor intervals in response to pharmacologic therapy, and assess for other arrhythmias.

Transthoracic Echocardiogram (TTE)

Determine LV size and function, screen for valvular and pericardial disease, measure atrial size, assess for LVH, and estimate pulmonary pressure. The sensitivity for detection of LA thrombus is low for TTE as opposed to TEE.

Laboratory Tests

Tests include thyroid panel, serum electrolytes, complete blood count (CBC), renal and hepatic function, and coagulation tests in part to assess for possible risk factors for AF and to guide pharmacologic therapy.

Additional tests may be indicated. This notably may include but is not limited to the following:

1. *Chest imaging*
2. *Holter monitoring or event recording* (in part to assess rate control, confirm diagnosis of AF, assess concomitant arrhythmias, and correlate symptoms)
3. *Exercise testing* (in part to evaluate for ischemia prior to using Class 1C antiarrhythmic drugs, assess rate control, define exercise tolerance, and possibly reproduce exercise-induced AF)

MANAGEMENT—OVERALL STRATEGY

While the management of patients with AF is highly individualized, principal components include the following:

1. Carefully consider and address the potential etiologies, risk factors, and/or triggers for AF
2. Control the ventricular rate, if needed
3. Initiate appropriate antithrombotic therapy, if safe, based primarily on assessment of overall stroke risk
4. Consider employing measures to restore and maintain sinus rhythm, if indicated, generally via cardioversion and antiarrhythmic drugs. If the patient's condition is unstable, urgent cardioversion should be performed.

Specific guidelines regarding each of these components are discussed in depth for the remainder of the chapter.

In all stable patients with atrial fibrillation of any clinical pattern, it is recommended that they be started on appropriate *antithrombotic therapy* (if safe) and *rate control* (if needed). However, the issue of whether or not attempts should also be made to *maintain sinus rhythm* is debatable. Despite the hypothesized benefits of maintaining sinus rhythm over rate control alone, randomized clinical trials comparing these two strategies have failed to show a statistically significant difference in mortality, stroke, or quality of life (see "Landmark Clinical Trials" section for further details).[7–11] Importantly, regardless of the strategy pursued, appropriate antithrombotic therapy is generally warranted.

MANAGEMENT—RATE CONTROL

Acute Setting

* The goal for the ventricular rate will vary significantly depending upon the clinical scenario.
* As outlined below, amiodarone may be an acceptable agent for rate control despite its multiple toxicities, if other measures are unsuccessful or contraindicated. The additional *antiarrhythmic* potential of amiodarone for facilitating conversion to sinus rhythm must be considered prior to use. (See Table 8-1.)

TABLE 8-1   Selected agents for rate control in the acute setting

Drug		Loading Dose	Maintenance Dose	Selected Side Effects and Comments
Patients without accessory pathways and no acute heart failure				
βB	Esmolol	0.5 mg/kg IV over 1 min; may repeat q 4 min while titrating IVCI	50–200 μg/kg/min IVCI	↓BP, HB, ↓HR, bronchospasm, HF; exercise extreme caution if used despite HF or hypotension though very short half-life
	Metoprolol	2.5 to 5 mg IV over 2 min; may repeat q 5 min up to 3 doses	No IVCI available	↓BP, HB, ↓HR, bronchospasm, HF; exercise extreme caution if used despite HF or hypotension
	Propranolol	0.15 mg/kg (~1 mg) IV q 2 min	No IVCI available	↓BP, HB, ↓HR, bronchospasm, HF; exercise extreme caution if used despite HF or hypotension
CCB	Diltiazem	0.25 mg/kg (~20 mg) IV over 2 min; may repeat in 15 min at dose of 0.35 mg/kg (~25 mg) IV over 2 min	5–15 mg/h IVCI	↓BP, HB, HF; exercise extreme caution if used despite HF or hypotension
	Verapamil	0.075 to 0.15 mg/kg (~5–10 mg) IV over 2 min; may repeat in 15–30 min	0.125 mg/min IVCI	↓BP, HB, HF; exercise extreme caution if used despite HF or hypotension

Patients with accessory pathway: Rate control may be appropriate though conversion to sinus rhythm and/or catheter ablation of the accessory pathway is generally recommended. Agents that slow conduction across the A-V node (including nondihydropyridine CCB, β-blockers, and digoxin) are not recommended as they may lead to rapid antegrade conduction across the accessory pathway during AF.

(continued)

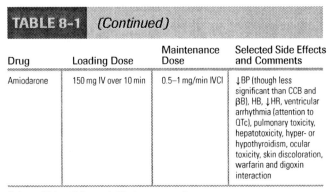

TABLE 8-1 *(Continued)*

Drug	Loading Dose	Maintenance Dose	Selected Side Effects and Comments
Amiodarone	150 mg IV over 10 min	0.5–1 mg/min IVCI	↓BP (though less significant than CCB and βB), HB, ↓HR, ventricular arrhythmia (attention to QTc), pulmonary toxicity, hepatotoxicity, hyper- or hypothyroidism, ocular toxicity, skin discoloration, warfarin and digoxin interaction

Patients with heart failure and without accessory pathway

Drug	Loading Dose	Maintenance Dose	Selected Side Effects and Comments
Digoxin	0.25 mg IV; may repeat cautiously q 2 h up to 1.5 mg (reduce dosage if used in renal insufficiency)	0.125–0.375 mg IV or PO daily (reduce dosage if used in renal insufficiency)	Digitalis toxicity, HB, ↓HR, amiodarone interaction; the onset of digoxin is slow (over 60 min or greater)
Amiodarone	150 mg IV over 10 min	0.5–1 mg/min IVCI	(see above)

Consult pharmacopoeia/manufacturer recommendations for most accurate and complete listings, and for additional appropriate drugs.
↓BP, hypotension; IVCI, intravenous continuous infusion; HB, heart block; HF, heart failure; ↓HR, bradycardia; NA, not applicable; and QTc, corrected QT interval
Modified from Fuster et al. ACC/AHA/ESC 2006 guidelines for the management of patients with atrial fibrillation. *Circulation.* 2006;114:700–752.[6]

Chronic Setting

* It is reasonable to pursue a goal ventricular rate of 60 to 80 bpm at rest and 90 to 115 bpm during moderate exercise.
* It is reasonable to consider using a 24-hour Holter monitor (with a goal overall average rate of approximately ≤100 bpm) and/or exercise testing as an adjunct in assessing the adequacy of rate control therapy.
* In selected patients with symptomatic, medically refractory atrial fibrillation, nonpharmacologic attainment of rate control via catheter ablation of the A-V node in conjunction with permanent ventricular pacing has been demonstrated to be effective and is associated with improvement in symptoms.[12]

See Table 8-2.

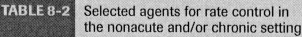

TABLE 8-2 Selected agents for rate control in the nonacute and/or chronic setting

Drug	Dosing Regimen	Onset	Major Side Effects and Comments
Metoprolol	25–100 mg PO twice a day	4–6 h	↓BP, HB, ↓HR, bronchospasm, HF
Propranolol	80–240 mg PO total daily, divided in 2–4 doses per day	60–90 min	↓BP, HB, ↓HR, bronchospasm, HF
Diltiazem	120–360 mg PO total daily, in divided doses depending upon formulation	2–4 h	↓BP, HB, HF
Verapamil	120–360 mg PO total daily, in divided doses depending upon formulation	1–2 h	↓BP, HB, HF, digoxin interaction
Amiodarone	Multiple dosing regimens are possible. One example is to load (in divided doses) with 800 mg PO daily for 1 wk, then 600 mg PO daily for 1 wk, then 400 mg PO daily for 4–6 wk, then 200 mg PO daily as maintenance dose	Days	↓BP (though less significant than CCB and βB), HB, ↓HR, ventricular arrhythmia (attention to QTc), pulmonary toxicity, hepatotoxicity, hyper- or hypothyroidism, ocular toxicity, skin discoloration, warfarin and digoxin interaction
Digoxin	May load with 0.5 mg PO daily up to 1.5 mg, then 0.125–0.375 mg daily as maintenance dose (reduce dosage if used in renal insufficiency)	2 days	Digitalis toxicity, HB, ↓HR, amiodarone interaction; consider monitoring digoxin serum levels. Not recommended as sole agent for rate control in paroxysmal AF.

Consult pharmacopoeia/manufacturer recommendations for most accurate and complete listings, and for additional appropriate drugs.
↓BP, hypotension; IVCI, intravenous continuous infusion; HB, heart block; HF, heart failure; ↓HR, brady-cardia; NA, not applicable; and QTc, corrected QT interval
Modified from Fuster et al. ACC/AHA/ESC 2006 guidelines for the management of patients with atrial fibrillation. *Circulation*. 2006;114:700–752.[6]

MANAGEMENT—RHYTHM CONTROL

Restoring Sinus Rhythm

Direct-current (DC) cardioversion is generally more effective and reliable than pharmacologic cardioversion and is typically preferred. The primary disadvantage of DC cardioversion is the requirement for conscious sedation or anesthesia. Pharmacologic cardioversion is an acceptable option in some scenarios, including for recent-onset AF (especially <48 hours).

- Direct-Current Cardioversion

  ○ Immediate DC cardioversion (as initial therapy or promptly after failed pharmacologic therapy) is suggested in unstable individuals, including those with symptomatic hypotension, myocardial ischemia, heart failure, or accessory pathways associated with hemodynamic compromise and/or rapid ventricular rate.

  ○ See section entitled "Management—Antithrombotic Therapy" for suggested anticoagulation therapy.

  ○ Pretreatment with some antiarrhythmic drugs may increase the likelihood of successful DC cardioversion, reduce the energy requirement needed for DC cardioversion, and enhance the likelihood of maintaining sinus rhythm.

  ○ The patient should be fasting with electrolytes and drug levels (including digoxin) within normal limits.

  ○ DC cardioversion should be *synchronized* to the R-wave. Although the required energy is variable and may need to be adjusted, it may be reasonable to use $\geq 200\,J$ monophasic (or $200\,J$ biphasic) as the initial shock for external cardioversion in most patients, based on higher rates of cardioversion.[13]

  ○ The operating team should be equipped for cardiopulmonary resuscitation. Prophylactic pacing measures should be available, especially in individuals with conduction system disease including sick sinus syndrome who are at risk for prolonged asystole or bradycardia following cardioversion.

- Pharmacologic Cardioversion

  ○ Although facilitation of cardioversion with medications increases the probability of restoring sinus rhythm, the spontaneous rate of cardioversion for recent-onset AF (especially within 24 hours) is greater than 50% in some series.[14]

  ○ Class IC drugs, such as propafenone and flecainide, are thought to be more effective than agents such as amiodarone (Class III) in effecting cardioversion for recent-onset AF. However, Class IC agents are thought to be less effective than Class III agents for pharmacologic cardioversion if the AF episode has been present for more than 7 days.[15]

  ○ IV preparations are associated with greater success rates than oral preparations.

  ○ Of the wide array of pharmacologic agents available for cardioversion, five of the more studied and well proven agents are included in Table 8-3.

TABLE 8-3 Selected agents for cardioversion of AF of up to 7 days

Drug (Vaughan Williams Class)	Dosing Regimen	Selected Side Effects
Flecainide (Class 1C)	Oral: 200–300 mg IV: 1.5–3 mg/kg over 10–20 min	• ↓BP, atrial flutter with rapid ventricular rate (consider use with β-blocker or nondihydropyridine CCB) • Ventricular arrhythmia[a] (avoid if CAD, HTN with LVH, or CHF; see below)
Propafenone (Class 1C)	Oral: 600 mg IV: 1.5–2 mg/kg over 10–20 min	• ↓BP, atrial flutter with rapid ventricular rate (consider use with β-blocker or nondihydropyridine CCB) • Ventricular arrhythmia[a] (avoid if CAD, HTN with LVH, or CHF; see below)
Amiodarone (Class III)	Oral: Load 1.2–1.8 g per day in divided dose until 10 g total, then maintenance dose 200–400 mg daily IV: Load 5–7 mg/kg over 30–60 min then 0.5–1 mg/min IVCI	• ↓HR, HB, ↓HR, GI upset, constipation, phlebitis (IV), pulmonary toxicity, hepatotoxicity, hyper- or hypothyroidism, ocular toxicity, skin discoloration, warfarin and digoxin interaction • QT prolongation, torsade de pointes/ventricular arrhythmia (rare)[b] (see below)

(continued)

TABLE 8-3 (Continued)

Drug (Vaughan Williams Class)	Dosing Regimen	Selected Side Effects
Dofetilide (Class III)	Oral: 500 μg BID if creatinine clearance >60 mL/min (reduce dosage if used in renal insufficiency; contraindicated if creatinine clearance <20 mL/min)	• QT prolongation, torsade de pointes/ventricular arrhythmia[b] (see below) • Use restricted and need for continuous monitoring given significant risk of torsade de pointes • IV formulation not available in United States
Ibutilide (Class III)	IV: 1 mg over 10 min; may repeat 1 mg IV when necessary	• QT prolongation, torsade de pointes/ventricular arrhythmia[b] (see below) • Use restricted and need for continuous monitoring given significant risk of torsade de pointes

Consult pharmacopoeia/manufacturer recommendations for most accurate and complete listings, and for additional appropriate drugs.

↓BP hypotension; HB, heart block; HF, heart failure; ↓HR, bradycardia; HTN, hypertension; QTc, corrected QT interval; CAD, coronary artery disease; HTN, hypertension; LVH, left ventricular hypertrophy; CHF, congestive heart failure; GI, gastrointestinal.

[a]Factors that predispose one to ventricular proarrhythmia with Class IC agents include, but are not limited to, structural heart disease (including CAD, CHF, HTN with substantial LVH), QRS >120 ms, concomitant VT, depressed LV function, rapid ventricular response rate, rapid dose increase, high dose (drug accumulation), and addition of other drugs with negative inotropic properties.

[b]Factors that predispose one to ventricular proarrhythmia with Class III agents include, but are not limited to, QTc >460 ms, long QT interval syndrome, excessive QT lengthening after drug initiation, structural heart disease (notably, substantial LVH), depressed LV function, hypokalemia, hypomagnesemia, female sex, renal insufficiency, bradycardia, previous proarrhythmia, rapid dose increase, high dose (drug accumulation), and addition of other QT-prolonging drugs, diuretics, or drugs listed in http://www.torsades.org/. Modified from Fuster et al. ACC/AHA/ESC 2006 guidelines for the management of patients with atrial fibrillation. *Circulation.* 2006;114:700-752.[6]

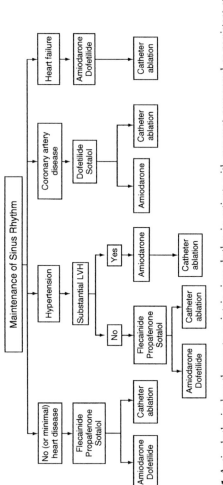

FIGURE 8-1 Antiarrhythmic drug therapy to maintain sinus rhythm in patients with recurrent paroxysmal or persistent atrial fibrillation. Within each box, drugs are listed alphabetically and not in order of suggested use. The vertical flow indicates order of preference under each condition. The seriousness of heart disease proceeds from left to right, and selection of therapy in patients with multiple conditions depends on the most serious condition present. LVH indicates left ventricular hypertrophy. (From Fuster et al. ACC/AHA/ESC 2006 guidelines for the management of patients with atrial fibrillation. *Circulation.* 2006;114:700–752.)[6]

Maintenance of Sinus Rhythm

Pharmacologic and nonpharmacologic options (including catheter ablation) are available if a strategy of rhythm control is attempted (Figure 8-1). Catheter ablation is not discussed here, as published long-term outcomes and larger trial data are lacking at present. However, it represents a promising treatment modality with a growing clinical experience. Although treatment decisions must be individualized, Figure 8-1 represents a framework for safely initiating therapy based on the proarrhythmic risks of these agents. Table 8-4 presents the maintenance dosing for some of the more commonly used agents. Drug guidelines must be consulted for safely initiating and monitoring antiarrhythmic therapy.

TABLE 8-4 Selected agents for maintenance of sinus rhythm

Drug	Total Daily Oral Dosage	Selected Side Effects
Flecainide	200–300 mg (generally divided in BID doses)	• ↓BP, atrial flutter with rapid ventricular rate (consider use with β-blocker or nondihydropyridine CCB) • Ventricular arrhythmia[a] (avoid if CAD, HTN with LVH, or CHF; see below)
Propafenone	450–900 mg (generally in divided doses depending upon formulation)	• ↓BP, atrial flutter with rapid ventricular rate (consider use with β-blocker or nondihydropyridine CCB) • Ventricular arrhythmia[a] (avoid if CAD, HTN with LVH, or CHF; see below)
Amiodarone	100–400 mg (generally preceded by loading regimen)	• ↓BP, HB, ↓HR, GI upset, constipation, phlebitis (IV), pulmonary toxicity, hepatotoxicity, hyper- or hypothyroidism, ocular toxicity, skin discoloration, warfarin and digoxin interaction • QT prolongation, (rare) torsade de pointes/ventricular arrhythmia[b] (see below)
Dofetilide	500–1000 μg (generally divided in BID doses); adjust dose for renal function and QT-interval response during in-hospital initiation phase	• QT prolongation, torsade de pointes/ventricular arrhythmia[b] (see below) • Use restricted and need for continuous monitoring given significant risk of torsade de pointes • IV formulation not available in United States

Drug	Total Daily Oral Dosage	Selected Side Effects
Sotalol	160–320 mg (generally in divided doses); adjust dose for renal function and QT-interval response; often requires in-hospital initiation phase	• QT prolongation, torsade de pointes/ventricular arrhythmia[b] (see below) • Additionally with β-blocking properties including exacerbation of bronchospastic disease

Consult pharmacopoeia/manufacturer recommendations for most accurate and complete listings, and for additional appropriate drugs.

↓BP, hypotension; HB, heart block; HF, heart failure; ↓HR, bradycardia; HTN, hypertension; QTc, corrected QT interval; CAD, coronary artery disease; HTN, hypertension; LVH, left ventricular hypertrophy; CHF, congestive heart failure; GT, gastrointestinal

[a]Factors that predispose one to ventricular proarrhythmia with Class IC agents include, but are not limited to, structural heart disease (including CAD, CHF, HTN with substantial LVH), QRS >120 ms, concomitant VT, depressed LV function, rapid ventricular response rate, rapid dose increase, high dose (drug accumulation), and addition of other drugs with negative inotropic properties.

[b]Factors that predispose one to ventricular proarrhythmia with Class III agents include, but are not limited to, QTc >460 ms, long QT interval syndrome, excessive QT lengthening after drug initiation, structural heart disease (notably, substantial LVH), depressed LV function, hypokalemia, hypomagnesemia, female sex, renal insufficiency, bradycardia, previous proarrhythmia, rapid dose increase, high dose (drug accumulation), and addition of other QT-prolonging drugs, diuretics, or drugs listed in http://www.torsades.org/.

Modified from Fuster et al. ACC/AHA/ESC 2006 guidelines for the management of patients withatrial fibrillation. *Circulation.* 2006;114:700–752.[6]

MANAGEMENT—ANTITHROMBOTIC THERAPY

Risk Factors for Ischemic Stroke and Systemic Embolism in AF

See Table 8-5.

 TABLE 8-5   Risk factors for ischemic stroke and systemic embolism in AF

Less Validated or Weaker Risk Factors	Moderate-risk Factors	High-risk Factors
Female sex	Age ≥75 y	Previous stroke, transient ischemic attack (TIA), or embolism
Age 65–74 y	Hypertension	Mitral stenosis
Coronary artery disease	Heart failure	Prosthetic heart valve
Thyrotoxicosis	Left ventricular (LV) ejection fraction ≤35% Diabetes mellitus	Hypertrophic cardiomyopathy

Modified from Fuster et al. ACC/AHA/ESC 2006 guidelines for the management of patients with atrial fibrillation. *Circulation.* 2006;114:700–752.[6]

Long-term Antithrombotic Therapy Guidelines

Decisions regarding appropriate antithrombotic therapy in patients with AF must be *individualized* based on overall risk versus benefit of therapy with specific attention to (a) assessment of one's overall stroke risk, (b) assessment of one's bleeding risk, and (c) patient preference, including ability to comply with proposed therapy. Notably, current practice places less emphasis on guiding decisions regarding antithrombotic therapy based on the pattern of AF—that is, paroxysmal, persistent, or permanent. Unless contraindications exist, antithrombotic therapy is generally recommended in all individuals with AF unless they have lone AF. Despite considerable debate among providers, particularly regarding individuals at intermediate risk for stroke, a framework for individualizing decisions based on assessment of stroke risk (see Table 8-5) is presented in Table 8-6.

ANTICOAGULATION IN SPECIAL POPULATIONS/SCENARIOS

Electrical or Pharmacologic Cardioversion

* In patients with AF episode of *known duration <48 hours* undergoing cardioversion, thromboembolic risk is mitigated, though present; whether or not antithrombotic therapy is needed must be individualized and is in part based on assessment of stroke risk.

* In patients with AF for *≥ 48 hours or of unknown duration*:

  ○ In hemodynamically *unstable* patients, cardioversion should be performed immediately with concomitant administration of IV heparin (if not contraindicated). At least 4 weeks of anticoagulation is suggested

TABLE 8-6 Antithrombotic therapy in AF

Risk Category (See Table 8-5)	Suggested Therapy
No risk factors	Aspirin (81–325 mg PO daily); need for aspirin is unclear though if lone AF and <60 y
One moderate risk factor (or ≥1 less validated/weaker risk factor, though more debated)	Aspirin (81–325 mg PO daily), or warfarin (INR 2–3 with target 2.5)
Any high-risk factor or more than 1 moderate risk factor	Warfarin (INR 2–3 with target 2.5); if a mechanical prosthesis is present, the INR should be at least ≥2.5 depending upon the prosthesis

Modified from Fuster et al. ACC/AHA/ESC 2006 guidelines for the management of patients with atrial fibrillation. *Circulation.* 2006;114:700–752.[6]

following successful cardioversion due to persistent thromboembolic risk, in part related to slow return of mechanical function ("stunning") of the left atrium (LA) and left atrium appendage (LAA). Given the propensity of AF to recur, prolonged anticoagulation following cardioversion is often advisable.

○ In hemodynamically *stable* patients, one may consider either (a) the conventional approach of empiric anticoagulation with warfarin for at least 3 weeks preceding cardioversion (with strict documentation of consistent therapeutic INR values between 2 and 3) or (b) a TEE-guided approach.[19] For further details describing these two approaches, refer to Figure 8-2 as well as the "Landmark Trials" section. In either scenario, a minimum of 4 weeks of anticoagulation is suggested following successful cardioversion.

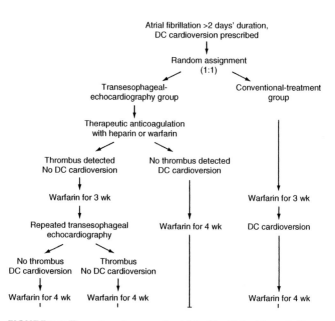

FIGURE 8-2 Figure 1 study protocol published by Klein AL, et al. (From Klein AL, Grimm RA, Murray RD, et al. Use of transesophageal echocardiography to guide cardioversion in patients with atrial fibrillation. *N Engl J Med.* 2001;344:1411–1420.)

Surgical or Diagnostic Procedures Associated with Bleeding Risk

In patients without high-risk for stroke (notably including mechanical prosthetic heart valve; see Table 8-5), it may be reasonable to interrupt anticoagulation for up to 1 week without using heparin.

Percutaneous Coronary Intervention

No clear data exist to guide optimal therapy. One potentially reasonable strategy is to use warfarin and clopidogrel for maintenance therapy with duration depending upon the type of stent implanted (aspirin may be added acutely until the INR is therapeutic); again, in the absence of data, this is an area of considerable debate and variability in practice.

LANDMARK CLINICAL TRIALS

See Tables 8-7 and 8-8.

TABLE 8-7   Rate versus rhythm control in AF

Trial	Details	Results/Comments
AFFIRM[7]	• 4,060 patients with paroxysmal or persistent AF; average f/u 3.5 y • Patients ≥65 y/o (mean age 69.7) with other risk factors for stroke or death (70.8% with hypertension) • Myriad antiarrhythmic interventions, though amiodarone most common (used by 62.8% in rhythm control at some point)	• Primary endpoint of overall mortality comparable: 26.7% in rhythm control vs. 25.9% in rate control ($p = 0.08$) • Rate of ischemic stroke comparable: 7.1% in rhythm control vs. 5.5% in rate control ($p = 0.79$) • Majority of strokes occurred in individuals who discontinued warfarin or had subtherapeutic INR; more individuals in rhythm control group discontinued warfarin
RACE[8]	• 522 patients with persistent AF or atrial flutter; average f/u 2.3 y • Mean age 68 y/o	• Primary composite endpoint of cardiovascular (CV) death, HF, thromboembolic complications, bleeding, pacemaker implantation, and severe adverse drug reaction comparable: 17.2% in rate control vs. 22.6% in rhythm control (90% confidence interval of −11 to 0.4%)
PIAF[9]	• 252 patients with persistent AF; average f/u 1 y • Mean age 61 y/o • Diltiazem first-line agent in rate control group; amiodarone first-line agent in rhythm control group	• Primary endpoint of improvement in symptoms related to AF comparable: 60.8% in rate control vs. 55.1% in rhythm control ($p = 0.317$)

Trial	Details	Results/Comments
HOT CAFÉ[10]	• 205 patients with first clinically overt episode of AF; average f/u 1.7 y • Mean age 60.8 y/o	• Primary composite endpoint of death, thromboembolic events, and major bleeding comparable: <5 events in each group with odds ratio between rate and rhythm control of 1.98 ($p > 0.71$)
STAF[11]	• 200 patients with persistent AF; average f/u 1.6 y • Mean age 66	• Primary composite endpoint of death, cardiopulmonary resuscitation, cerebrovascular event and systemic embolus comparable: 5.54% per year in rhythm control vs. 6.09% per year in rate control ($p = 0.99$)

TABLE 8-8 **Antithrombotic strategies in AF**

Strategy	Comments/Findings
Adjusted-dose warfarin vs. placebo: meta-analysis[16]	• Six trials using an intention-to-treat analysis of 2,900 patients with nonvalvular AF • 62% overall relative RR of stroke with warfarin (95% CI of 48%–72%); statistically significant in 4 of 6 individual trials • 2.7% per year absolute RR of stroke with warfarin in the five *primary* prevention trials analyzed (to prevent 1 stroke per year, NNT = 37) • 8.4% per year absolute relative risk (RR) of stroke with warfarin in the one *secondary* prevention trial analyzed (NNT = 12) • Nine total intracranial hemorrhages among the 2,900 patients (6 in the warfarin group [0.3% per year] vs. 3 in the placebo group [0.1% per year]; not statistically significantly different) • Significantly more extracranial hemorrhages per year in the warfarin group (0.9%) compared to the placebo group (0.6%) in the 5 studies included for analysis • Significant reduction in all-cause mortality with warfarin • Caveat that these clinical trials excluded patients at high risk for bleeding, and, as opposed to actual clinical practice, involved generally shorter time of follow-up (mean 1.6 y), younger patients (mean 69 y), and more stringent monitoring of anticoagulation
Aspirin vs. placebo: meta-analysis[16]	• Six trials using an intention-to-treat analysis of 3,337 patients with nonvalvular AF • 22% overall relative RR of stroke with aspirin (95% CI of 2%–38%)

(continued)

TABLE 8-8 *(Continued)*

Strategy	Comments/Findings
	• 1.5% per year absolute RR of stroke with aspirin for *primary* prevention (NNT = 67) • 2.5% per year absolute RR of stroke with aspirin for *secondary* prevention (NNT = 40) • No significant differences between intracranial hemorrhage, extracranial hemorrhage, nor mortality • Caveat: Modest benefit for stroke prevention with aspirin in this meta-analysis questioned due to (a) favorable results being largely driven by the Stroke Prevention in Atrial Fibrillation (SPAF) study,[17] the only trial of the six demonstrating a statistically significant benefit with aspirin therapy; and (b) apparent statistically significant advantage of aspirin in nondisabling stroke only, and not disabling stroke, per a subanalysis of the three largest trials reporting data on stroke severity
Aspirin AND Clopidogrel vs. vitamin K antagonist ACTIVE W[18]	• 3,335 patients with AF and ≥1 stroke risk factor randomized to clopidogrel 75 mg QD + aspirin 75–100 mg QD versus oral anticoagulation with vitamin K antagonist (VKA) • Trial stopped prematurely given evidence of clear superiority of VKA in reducing the primary composite outcome of stroke, non-CNS systemic embolic event, MI, and vascular death (3.93% annual risk with VKA vs. 5.6% with clopidogrel + ASA; $p = 0.0003$) • Major bleeding rates not significantly different • Separate question examining the role of dual antiplatelet therapy versus aspirin monotherapy in patients unable or unwilling to take warfarin currently being studied in the ACTIVE A arm
Use of TEE to guide duration of anticoagulation prior to elective cardioversion in patients with AF[19]	• (see preceding text for flow sheet of study design) • In 1,222 patients with AF for >2 d scheduled for elective cardioversion, comparable safety of a conventional approach (3 wk empiric anticoagulation with warfarin) to a TEE-guided approach (cardioversion performed shortly after brief anticoagulation therapy *if* patients with no detected thrombi): composite primary end point of CVA, TIA, and peripheral embolism within 8 wk was 0.8% in TEE group vs. 0.5% in conventional-treatment group ($p = 0.50$) • In TEE group, significantly lower hemorrhage rate (2.9%) than in the conventional approach, (5.5%, $p = 0.03$)

REFERENCES

1. Thom T, Haase N, Rosamond W, et al. American Heart Association. Heart disease and stroke statistics: 2006 Update. *Circulation.* 2006;113:85–151.
2. Lloyd-Jones DM, Wang TJ, Leip EP, et al. Lifetime risk for development of atrial fibrillation. *Circulation.* 2004;110:1042–1046.
3. Haissaguerre M, Jais P, Shah DC, et al. Spontaneous initiation of atrial fibrillation by ectopic beats originating in the pulmonary veins. *N Engl J Med.* 1998;339:659–666.
4. Olgin JE, Zipes DP. Specific arrhythmias: Diagnosis and treatment. In: Zipes DP, Libby P, Bonow RO, Braunwald E, eds. *Braunwald's Heart Disease: A Textbook of Cardiovascular Medicine,* 7th ed. Philadelphia: Elsevier Saunders;2005:803–863.
5. Wolf PA, Abbott RD, Kannell WB. Atrial fibrillation as an independent risk factor for stroke: The Framingham Study. *Stroke.* 1991;22:983–988.
6. Fuster V, Ryden LE, Cannom DS, et al. ACC/AHA/ESC 2006 guidelines for the management of patients with atrial fibrillation: A report of the American College of Cardiology/American Heart Association Task Force on Practice Guidelines and the European Society of Cardiology Committee for Practice Guidelines (Writing Committee to Revise the 2001 Guidelines for the Management of Patients With Atrial Fibrillation). *Circulation* 2006;114:e257–e354.
7. Wyse DG, Waldo AL, DiMarco JP, et al. Atrial fibrillation follow-up investigation of rhythm management (AFFIRM) investigators. A comparison of rate control and rhythm control in patients with atrial fibrillation. *N Engl J Med.* 2002;347:1825–1833.
8. Van Gelder IC, Hagens VE, Bosker HA, et al., for the Rate Control versus Electrical Cardioversion for Persistent Atrial Fibrillation Study Group (RACE). A comparison of rate control and rhythm control in patients with recurrent persistent atrial fibrillation. *N Engl J Med.* 2002;347:1834–1840.
9. Hohnloser SH, Kuck KH, Lilienthal J, for the PIAF Investigators. Rhythm or rate control in atrial fibrillation—pharmacological intervention in atrial fibrillation (PIAF): A randomized trial. *Lancet.* 2000;356:1789–1794.
10. Opolski G, Torbicki A, Kosior DA, et al. Rate control vs. rhythm control in patients with nonvalvular persistent atrial fibrillation: The results of the Polish How to Treat Chronic Atrial Fibrillation (HOT CAFÉ) study. *Chest.* 2004;126:476–486.
11. Carlsson J, Miketic S, Windeler J, et al., for the STAF Investigators. Randomized trial of rate-control versus rhythm-control in persistent atrial fibrillation: The Strategies of Treatment of Atrial Fibrillation (STAF) study. *J Am Coll Cardiol.* 2003;41:1690–1696.

12. Wood MA, Brown-Mahoney C, Kay GN, et al. Clinical outcomes after ablation and pacing therapy for atrial fibrillation. *Circulation.* 2000;101:1138–1144.

13. Joglar JA, Hamdan MH, Ramaswamy K, et al. Initial energy for elective external cardioversion of persistent atrial fibrillation. *Am J Cardiol.* 2000;86:348–350.

14. Hersi A, Wyse G. Medical management of atrial fibrillation. *Curr Cardiol Rep.* 2006;8:323–329.

15. Rudo T, Kowey P. Atrial fibrillation: Choosing an antiarrhythmic drug. *Curr Cardiol Rep.* 2006;8:370–376.

16. Hart RG, Benavente O, McBride R, et al. Antithrombotic therapy to prevent stroke in patients with atrial fibrillation: A meta-analysis. *Ann Intern Med.* 1999;131:492–501.

17. Stroke Prevention in Atrial Fibrillation (SPAF) investigators. Stroke Prevention in Atrial Fibrillation study. Final results. *Circulation.* 1991:84:527–539.

18. The ACTIVE Writing Group. Clopidogrel plus aspirin versus oral anticoagulation for atrial fibrillation in the atrial fibrillation clopidogrel trial with irbesartan for prevention of vascular events (ACTIVE W): A randomized controlled trial. *Lancet.* 2006:367:1903–1912.

19. Klein AL, Grimm RA, Murray RD, et al. Use of transesophageal echocardiography to guide cardioversion in patients with atrial fibrillation. *N Engl J Med.* 2001;344:1411–1420.

CHAPTER 9

Heart Failure

DAVID KAO, DAVID V. DANIELS, AND EUAN ASHLEY

BACKGROUND AND APPROACH

Approximately 5 million people throughout the United States have heart failure (HF); 550,000 are diagnosed each year, and it represents the primary diagnosis in over 1 million hospitalizations annually.[1,2] We will focus our efforts on the recognition and management of HF as an inpatient problem with the understanding that encounters may be prompted by everything from new onset HF, decompensation of patients with known HF, to refractory HF. We will make recommendations on reasonable strategies of acute HF management and initialization of chronic therapies known to have long-term benefit in terms of morbidity and mortality.

DEFINITION

Failure of the heart to pump blood forward at a sufficient rate to meet the metabolic demands of peripheral tissues, or the ability to do so only at the expense of abnormally high cardiac filling pressures.[3]

CLINICAL PRESENTATIONS OF HEART FAILURE

See Table 9-1.

Type

* Up to 44% isolated diastolic dysfunction, often mixed diastolic and systolic dysfunction

Systolic Dysfunction

* Most commonly secondary to ischemic heart disease (50%–75%) or primary valvular disease
* Differential diagnosis for nonischemic dilated cardiomyopathy (DCM) is very broad including toxins, medications, autoimmune, viral and bacterial infection, nutritional, familial, endocrine, pregnancy, isolated ventricular noncompaction

Diastolic Dysfunction

* Associated most commonly with chronic hypertension (HTN), left ventricular hypertrophy (LVH), and metabolic syndrome
* Infiltrative etiologies include hemochromatosis, sarcoidosis, and amyloidosis
* Can be seen acutely with ischemia as well as chronic coronary artery disease (CAD) after multiple myocardial infarctions (MI)

TABLE 9-1	Clinical presentations of heart failure	
Volume overload	Acute pulmonary edema	Low output state
• Gradual worsening of symptoms • Increased weight, edema • Dyspnea increased often with minimal pulmonary edema • Signs of right-sided volume overload often present including ↑ JVP, peripheral edema, ascites, pleural effusions • Elevated creatinine often improves with diuresis	• Acute dyspnea at rest • Generally hypoxemic respiratory failure • Often older patients, women > men, isolated diastolic function common • Triggers can be med noncompliance, pain, infection/fevers, or dietary indiscretions • Significant and hypertension and high catecholamine state common • Frank pulmonary edema often on CXR • Often not totally body volume overloaded and neck veins may not be elevated • Generally responds quickly to CPAP/BIPAP and vasodilator therapy with minimal diuresis	• Signs of hypoperfusion including relative hypotension, altered mentation, azotemia, oliguria, cool extremities • Generally severely impaired ejection fraction • May be volume overloaded or rarely intravascularly depleted and in a low output state as a result of overdiuresis • Invasive hemodynamics may have a role in diagnosis and stabilization • Often requires positive inotropic or vasodilator therapy

COMMON CAUSES OF ACUTE ON CHRONIC EXACERBATIONS

Forgotten meds (most common cause)
Anemia/Arrhythmias
Ischemia/Infection
Lifestyle (dietary indiscretion, non-steroidal anti-inflammatories [NSAID])
Upregulation of cardiac output (e.g., thyrotoxicosis, cocaine)
Renal failure
Embolism (PE)

HISTORY

- Recent chest pains (CP) or symptoms of ischemia
- Recent palpitations
- History of congestive heart failure (CHF), CAD, HTN
- Prior cardiac workup (i.e., echo, stress test, cardiac catheterizations)
- Functional status/exercise capacity (e.g., flights of stairs or number of blocks before having to rest)
- Changes in weight (e.g., clothes or rings not fitting recently), dependent edema, nocturia, paroxysmal nocturnal dyspnea (PND), orthopnea (most sensitive symptom of elevated pulmonary capillary wedge pressure (PCWP))[1]
- Recent changes in medications or missed doses—be specific about timing
- Recent changes in eating habits such as dining out, special events (e.g., holidays and weddings)

PHYSICAL EXAM

SIGNS OF RIGHT VENTRICULAR (RV) FAILURE

- Elevated jugular venous pressure (JVP) or + hepatojugular reflex
- Hepatomegaly or pulsatile liver
- Dependent peripheral edema
- Ascites
- Parasternal heave
- S3 or S4 at lower R sternal edge

SIGNS OF LEFT VENTRICULAR (LV) FAILURE

- Tachypnea, diaphoresis
- Enlarged or displaced point of maximal impulse (PMI)
- Early inspiratory rales (often not present in chronic failure) and hypoxemia
- Decreased breath sounds with decreased tactile fremitus at lung bases
- S3 (specific if present but not very sensitive) or summation gallop
- Murmur/thrill suggestive of severe valvular regurgitation or septal defect

SIGNS OF LOW CARDIAC OUTPUT

* Cool extremities
* Oliguria
* Altered mental status
* Narrow pulse pressure (pulse pressure <25% of the systolic blood pressure (SBP) has a sensitivity and specificity of 91% and 83% for a cardiac index of <2.2 L/min/m^2)[4]
* Tachypnea with normal oxygen saturation
* Pulsus alternans (ominous)

LABORATORY EXAMS AND IMAGING

CARDIAC ENZYMES

* Always exclude ischemia/infarct as etiology of acute HF
* Rule out with serial enzymes, as in acute myocardial infarction (AMI)
* Low-grade troponin may be detectable and even expected with significantly elevated left ventricular end diastolic pressure (LVEDP), CKMB often negative, and enzymes do not follow the typical rise and fall seen in an acute coronary syndrome

CREATININE AND THE CARDIO-RENAL SYNDROME

* Chronic renal failure is often associated with CHF, termed the "cardio-renal syndrome"
* Acute renal failure often due to further worsening of cardiac output
* Remember that decreased cardiac output (CO) is one cause of prerenal azotemia
* Rising creatinine during treatment of acute HF is associated with worse in-hospital and long-term outcomes
* Often "volume overload" presentations associated with creatinine improvement in the face of diuresis . . . ? Improved CO versus lowering venous back pressure/congestion on kidneys

B-TYPE NATRIURETIC PEPTIDE (BNP)

* Most useful for *excluding* CHF as a contributor to clinical presentation
* >150 pg/mL had a sensitivity and specificity of 85% and 83% and LR (+) of 5.3, LR (−) 0.18 for the diagnosis of heart failure in the Breathing Not Properly trial[3]
* Elevated BNP in the setting of intact systolic function (nl EF) is highly suggestive of diastolic dysfunction[5]
* BNP >400 pg/mL is virtually diagnostic of LV failure contributing to symptoms[6]

- May be normal in cases of restrictive or constrictive physiology
- Use caution in interpreting test in patients with chronic renal insufficiency (CRI), where brain natriuretic peptide (BNP) elevation may be exaggerated
- Pro-NT BNP had a higher cutoff but similar operating characteristics[7]:
  - Optimal cutoff for age:
  - $<50 = 450\,\text{pg/mL}$
  - 50 to 75 = 900 pg/mL
  - $>75 = 1800\,\text{pg/mL}$
  - above cutoffs yield a sensitivity of 90%, specificity of 84%

URINE TOXICOLOGY
- Rule out cocaine or amphetamine use as an etiology of heart failure in suspected patients

ECG
- Useful for rapidly detecting ST segment elevation MI (STEMI) as a cause of new onset HF but beware "strain" can be an effect of HF
- Arrhythmias such as A fib or high-grade A-V block as a precipitant of HF
- Q waves and left bundle branch block (LBBB) are good predictors of systolic dysfunction. QRS >220 milliseconds portends a poor prognosis
- Nonspecific intraventricular conduction delay >160 milliseconds suggests cardiomyopathy

CHEST X-RAY
- May demonstrate pulmonary edema, cardiomegaly, pleural effusions
- Useful for excluding other etiologies of symptoms
- If rapid change in heart size, consider pericardial effusion/tamponade

ECHO
- Universally the single most important test in the evaluation of new onset HF
- Rapidly differentiates among many etiologies listed above
- Can be difficult to identify restrictive or constrictive physiology
- Markers of diastolic dysfunction controversial and difficult in A fib

REST-STRESS ECHO, MRI OR PET SCANNING
- ALWAYS evaluate for ischemia in new-onset CHF, consider angiography as below
- Useful for assessing viability of myocardium and potential for response to revascularization
- Dobutamine echo may help determine response to aortic valve replacement (AVR) in critical aortic stenosis

PULMONARY ARTERY CATHETERIZATION
* May be helpful in titration of inotropes and vasodilators
* No benefit in large-scale randomized trials

CORONARY ANGIOGRAPHY
* Definitely if evidence of acute ischemia/infarct as cause of HF
* Consider in newly diagnosed systolic dysfunction as the gold standard for evaluation of coronary disease and potentially treatable lesions

CARDIOPULMONARY FUNCTIONAL VO$_2$ MAX TESTING
* Infrequently used in acute setting, can be useful for determining a cardiac or pulmonary cause of dyspnea when the etiology is unclear
* Used in severe HF in making objective assessments about transplantation

GENERAL APPROACH TO ACUTE MANAGEMENT OF HF

(See Figure 9-1.)

Pearls on Diuresis
* In a hemodynamically stable patient who is volume overloaded, your goal should be at least 1 to 2 liters/day
* In patients with renal insufficiency, consider continuous furosemide infusion rather than bolus dosing[8]

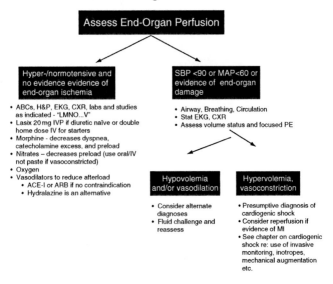

FIGURE 9-1 General approach to the acute management of HF.

- Strict I/Os and/or daily weights are essential to monitor diuresis
- Cardiac monitoring and frequent electrolyte checks (particularly magnesium and potassium) with aggressive replacement is essential to prevent arrhythmias
- Encourage the patient to take an active role by asking the nursing staff their weight daily
- Most patients respond to aggressive diuresis despite theoretical concerns of decreasing cardiac output
- Diuretics alone rarely cause serious hypotension
- Clinical deterioration with diuresis suggest preload-dependence such as severe pulmonary hypertension/RV failure, aortic stenosis, LV outflow tract obstruction, tamponade, constrictive pericarditis, or restrictive cardiomyopathy
- If diuresis is inadequate consider adding metolazone (limited data),[9] chlorothiazide, or nesiritide
- Double the dose when switching from IV to oral furosemide to achieve equivalent diuretic effect
- Consider oral bumetanide as an alternative to oral furosemide (better absorption in CHF but shorter elimination half-life)[10]

Noninvasive Positive Pressure Ventilation
- Consider continuous positive airway pressure (CPAP) as a bridge while diuresing and has recently been shown to have significant mortality benefit and decreases need for intubation in a large meta-analysis[11]
- Strongly consider in patients with increased work of breathing or persistent hypoxia despite initial therapy
- CPAP probably preferred to bilevel positive airway pressure (BIPAP) as there is some evidence of a trend toward increased AMI with BIPAP in comparison to CPAP[11]
- Reasonable to start with 8 cm H_2O and titrate to effect
- Contraindications: Inability to protect airway, craniofacial deformities limiting mask fit, hemodynamic instability, high oxygen requirement that cannot be achieved with BIPAP, nausea/vomiting due to risk of aspiration, and significant arrhythmias

SPECIFIC THERAPIES FOR SYSTOLIC DYSFUNCTION

GOALS
- Optimize preload, minimize afterload via vasodilator and diuretic therapy
- Prevent worsening of ejection fraction (EF) via ischemic events, tachyarrhythmia, excess afterload
- Reduce risk of life-threatening arrhythmia

ACE Inhibitors and ARBs
- Multiple trials that show mortality benefit (see below). ACE-I[12,13,14] or ARBs[15] > nitrates and hydralazine[16]

- ACE-Is are the preferred vasodilator and should be given a trial before hydralazine and nitrates
- Enalapril, losartan, and candesartan best studied, but presumed to be class-effect
- Start ACE-Is low and titrate while watching K and renal function closely
- The lower the EF, the more benefit from ACE-I/ARB if tolerated
- Allow for a 30% increase in creatinine with therapy before considering the patient intolerant

Hydralazine/Nitrates

- First vasodilator therapy to show survival benefit versus placebo[16]
- Subsequently found to be inferior to ACE-I/ARBs,[17] though best alternative for patients intolerant to ACE-I/ARB
- Goal dose in VHeFT-I: hydralazine 300 mg/day + 160 mg isosorbide dinitrate/day[16]
- May have an additive benefit to ACE-I/ARB, though only studied in self-identified "African descent" patients so far[18]

Beta Blockers

- Multiple trials show mortality benefit[19,20,21,22,23]
- Some patients may have dramatic improvement in EF with therapy
- Not all beta-blockers are created equal![24]

CHOICE OF AGENT

- Carvedilol (use caution in severe asthma because nonselective) > metoprolol succinate for increasing EF but both show mortality benefit[25]
- Metoprolol succinate (long acting) is the type of metoprolol best studied in CHF[25]
- Patients with low BP may tolerate metoprolol better and those who are hypertensive may get more BP-lowering effects from carvedilol[25]
- Metoprolol may worsen insulin resistance, carvedilol has neutral effect[26]
- Consider compliance when selecting regimen (once versus twice daily dosing—Coreg XR now available however)

INITIATION, TITRATION, AND SIDE EFFECTS

- Start at low dose if stable off inotrope therapy
- See landmark trials section below for starting doses in clinical trials
- Symptomatic benefit may take months and patients may complain of initial worsening of symptoms
- Titrate primarily as an outpatient, increase dose to highest tolerated by blood pressure (BP), heart rate (HR)
- Side effects include increased fatigue, hypotension, water retention, azotemia, decreased libido/impotence, theoretically exacerbation of reactive airway disease
- Consider maintaining beta blockade while intensifying diuresis in patients treated for >3 months with increased congestive symptoms

- Decrease or hold in patients presenting with severe acute-HF, especially with low output symptoms or significant azotemia

Aldosterone Antagonists (Spironolactone/Eplerenone)
- Indicated for NYHA class III-IV HF (RALES)[27] and post-MI heart failure (EPHESUS)
- Best-studied in patients *already on ACE-I or ARB*[27]
- Significant reduction in mortality and hospitalization[27]
- Contraindicated with K >5.0 mEq/L, Cr >2.5 mg/dL, or CrCl <30 mL/min
- Extreme caution in patients with Cr >1.5 mg/dL or CrCl <50 mL/min
- Also consider in patients with resistant hypokalemia on standard therapy
- Close monitoring for hyperkalemia is critical, especially in setting of CRI[28,29]
- Stop exogenous K replacement and monitor serum K and Cr at 3 days, 1 week, and monthly after initiation of therapy for at least the first 3 months
- Eplerenone is alternative to spironolactone that does not produce gynecomastia[30]

Digoxin
- May be considered after first-line therapies including RAAS inhibition, beta blockers, and aldosterone antagonists are maximized or in conjunction with A-V nodal agents for improving rate control in atrial fibrillation
- Can be considered as an adjunct especially in patients with AF with RVR, decreases hospitalizations and improves symptoms[31]
- Post hoc analysis of the DIG trial suggests serum dig concentration (SDC) of 0.5 to 0.8 ng/mL may be associated with mortality benefits as well[32]
- Consider no more than 0.125 mg daily in all patients
- Do not load unless being used as an adjunct for rate control
- Close attention to prevention of hypokalemia which can promote toxicities

Nesiritide
- Natriuretic that reduces preload and afterload without effect on contractility
- More rapid improvement in PCWP and dyspnea over placebo but similar when compared to nitroglycerin (NTG),[33] milrinone, or dobutamine[34]
- Clinically may be a useful adjunct to standard therapy in refractory HF and as bridge to transplant
- Optional 2 μg/kg bolus, followed by infusion at 0.01 to 0.03 μg/kg/min
- Less likely to promote ventricular arrhythmias compared to dobutamine[35]

Anticoagulation
- All patients with ischemic cardiomyopathy should at least be on aspirin[36]
- Patients in AF should be on Coumadin (INR 2.0–3.0) if there is no contraindication
- Those with severely depressed EF (<30%), large territory of akinetic LV, or evidence of LV thrombus probably benefit from anticoagulation as well[36]

Internal Cardioverter Defibrillators
• See chapter on sudden death

Revascularization Therapy
• Evaluate for contribution of ischemia; see chapter on CAD for indications and strategy.

TABLE 9-2	Heart failure treatment strategies checklist			
	Stage A; At risk for HF but no symptoms or structural abnormalities	Stage B; Structural heart disease *without* symptoms or signs of HF	Stage C; Structural heart disease *with* current or past symptoms of HF	Stage D; Refractory HF despite maximal conventional therapy
Aggressive BP control • Goal <130/80	X	X	X	X
Aggressive lipid management • Goal LDL <100 and <70 with CAD or DM • Statins generally preferred	X	X	X	X
Lifestyle modifications • Facilitate cessation of smoking, alcohol, illicit drugs • Emphasize importance of patient role in daily monitoring of status (e.g., weight, diet, symptoms) • Encourage exercise to the point of developing sx	X	X	X	X

	Stage A	Stage B	Stage C	Stage D
Avoid NSAIDS, calcium channel blockers, and antiarrhythmics except B-blockers • Aspirin OK, particularly if ischemic CM • Most antiarrhythmics a/w increased mortality except amiodarone and dofetilide • Calcium channel blockers a/w increased mortality in patients with ↓ EF except dihydropyridine which can be used as a BP control adjunct if other treatment maximized		X	X	X
Na restriction • *Goal*: <2 G Na per day • Refer to nutrionist, compliance very difficult			X	X
ACE Inhibitors/ARB • *Goal*: Highest dose tolerated by BP, RF but most benefit in low dose range • *Contraindications*: Cr >3.0, history of angioedema, prior episode of ARF with drug, or pregnancy • *Caution*: known bilateral RAS, SBP < 80 mm Hg, acute renal failure, K >5.5 meq/L	Consider in selected patients	Consider in selected patients	X	X

(continued)

TABLE 9-2 *(Continued)*				
	Stage A	Stage B	Stage C	Stage D
Beta-blockers • Metoprolol succinate or carvedilol best studied • *Goal*: Highest dose tolerated by BP, HR, side effect • *Caution*: HR <60, symptomatic hypotension, low output state, heart block, reactive airway disease especially with a significant reversible component		Consider in selected patients	X	X
Hydralazine/Nitrates • Alternative to ACE-I or ARB • May have value as adjunct to ACE-I/ARB • *Goal*: Highest doses tolerated by BP, sx • *Contraindications*: Use of PDE-5 inhibitors (e.g., Viagra)		Consider in selected patients	X	X
Aldosterone antagonists • Consider as adjunct to ACE-I/ARB • *Goal*: Spironolactone 25 mg or eplerenone 50 mg qd • *Caution*: Renal failure, hyperkalemia			X	X

	Stage A	Stage B	Stage C	Stage D
Loop diuretics • Cornerstone of volume, sx management • Bumetanide or torsemide an alternative to furosemide if concern for bowel edema			X	X
Digoxin • Consider as adjunct if first-line therapy insufficient • *Goal*: low dose ($\leq$0.125 mg daily, ideally to level 0.5-0.8 ng/ml) • Contraindicated with significant renal failure			Consider in select patients	Consider in selected patients
Nesiritide • Comparable to combined diuretics + NTG • *Goal*: 0.01-0.03 mcg/kg/min +/− 2 mcg/kg bolus • *Caution*: Hypotension, active ischemia			Consider in selected patients	Consider in selected patients

Heart Failure with a Normal EF and No Valvular Disease (Diastolic Dysfunction)

Not nearly as well studied and the jury is still out on optimal treatment.

Rate Control

* Attractive physiologically though yet unproven to alter end points clinically
* Carvedilol shown in one study to improve hemodynamics in diastolic HF[37]
* No hard end points studied

ACE-I

* Results from an analysis of the HOPE study suggests ACE-Is have beneficial effects on structure and function in patients with diastolic dysfunction and normal BP[38]

ARB

* See CHARM-Preserved below

Spironolactone
* Recent study suggests spironolactone improves hemodynamics in isolated diastolic HF,[39] though no hard end-point data yet

LANDMARK CLINICAL TRIALS

See Table 9-3.

TABLE 9-3	Landmark clinical trials related to heart failure	
Drug	**Trial and design**	**Results**
Digoxin	**DIG Trial** – *NEJM*, 1997[31] 6,800 pts – EF <45% in NSR *Digoxin 0.25 mg/d vs. placebo*	22% RRR of hospitalization **NNT = 13** No sig diff in all-cause mortality
	Digoxin level and outcomes in DIG Trial – *JAMA*, 2003[32] **Post hoc analysis stratified by dig level**	Dig level of 0.5-0.8 ng/mL: 28% RRR of death **NNT = 16**
Nitrates + hydralazine	**V-HeFT I** – *NEJM*, 1986[16] 642 men – NYHA 2-4 *Hydralazine 300 mg/d + isosorbide dinitrate 160 mg/d vs. prazosin 20 mg/d vs. placebo*	Mortality same in prazosin vs. placebo 34% RRR of death at 2, 3 y with H/N **NNT = 11 at 2 y, 9 at 3 y**
	A-HeFT – *NEJM*, 2004[18] 1,050 pts – NYHA 3-4 on "standard therapy" including ACE-I, ARB, or B-blockers x >3 mo *37.5-225 mg hydralazine + 20-120 mg isosorbide dinitrate vs. placebo*	Stopped early due to mortality benefit 40% RRR all-cause death **NNT = 25** 33% RRR of first CHF admit **NNT = 13**
Angiotensin-Converting-Enzyme Inhibitors	**CONSENSUS** – *NEJM*, 1987[13] 253 pts – NYHA class IV *Enalapril 2.5-40 mg/d vs. placebo*	27% RRR of death at 1 y **NNT = 7**
	SOLVD – *NEJM*, 1991[14] 2,569 pts – EF <35%, NYHA 2-3 *Enalapril 2.5-20 mg/d vs. placebo*	16% RRR of all-cause death **NNT = 25** 26% RRR of death/CHF admit **NNT = 10**

Drug	Trial and design	Results
Angiotensin-Converting-Enzyme Inhibitors (cont'd.)	**SOLVD** – *NEJM*, 1992[12] 4,228 pts – EF <35%, NYHA 1 *Enalapril 2.5-20 mg/d vs. placebo*	No mortality benefit RRR 37% of developing CHF **NNT = 10**
	V-HeFT II – *NEJM*, 1991[17] 804 men – NYHA 2-3 on dig/diuretics *Enalapril 20 mg/d vs. hydralazine 300 mg/d + isosorbide dinitrate 160 mg/d*	28% RRR of death at 2 y **NNT = 25** *Difference mostly in sudden death in pts with less severe sx*
Angiotensin Receptor Blockers	**ELITE** – *Lancet*, 1997[40] 722 pts – EF <40%, NYHA 2-4 *Losartan 50 mg/d vs. captopril 150 mg/d*	**8% ARR of d/c meds due to side effects** RRR 46% all-cause mortality **NNT = 25** (unexpected result!)
	ELITE II – *Lancet*, 2000[41] 3,152 pts – EF <40%, NYHA 2-4 *Losartan 50 mg/d vs. captopril 150 mg/d*	No difference in all-cause mortality **5% ARR of med d/c due to side effects**
	CHARM-Overall – *Lancet*, 2003[42] 7,601 pts – NYHA 2-4 x at least 4 weeks *Candesartan 4-32 mg/d vs. placebo*	No difference in all-cause death 18% RRR of CV death/admit **NNT = 23**
	CHARM-Added – *Lancet*, 2003[43] 2,548 pts – EF <40%, NYHA 2-4, already on ACE-inhibitor *Candesartan 4-32 mg/d vs. placebo*	No difference in all-cause death 15% RRR of CV death/admit **NNT = 23**
	CHARM-Alternative – *Lancet*, 2003[15] 2,028 pts – EF <40%, NYHA 2-4, intolerant of ACE-inhibitor *Candesartan 4-32 mg/d vs. placebo*	13% RRR of death **NNT = 33** 30% RRR for CV death/admit **NNT = 14**
	CHARM-Preserved – *Lancet*, 2003[44] 3,023 pts – EF >40%, NYHA 2-4 *Candesartan 4-32 mg/d vs. placebo*	RRR of all-cause death nonsignificant 16% RRR of admit for CHF **NNT = 41**

(continued)

TABLE 9-3	*(Continued)*	
Drug	**Trial and design**	**Results**
Angiotensin Receptor Blockers (cont'd.)	**VALHeFT** – *NEJM*, 2001[45] 5,010 pts – EF <40%, NYHA 2-4 on either diuretics, ACE-I, dig, B-blockers, or combo *Valsartan 160 mg bid vs. placebo*	No difference in all-cause death 13% RRR of death, cardiac arrest with resuscitation, CHF admit or output IV tx **NNT = 30** *Subgroup suggests RR of death 1.4 in pts on ACE-I and B-blockers*
Aldosterone antagonists	**RALES** – *NEJM*, 1999[27] 1,663 pts – EF <35%, NYHA III-IV, on diuretics (100%) and ACE-I (95%) *Spironolactone 25-50 mg/d vs. placebo*	Stopped early due to mortality benefit 30% RRR of death **NNT = 10** 10% men had gynecomastia/ breast pain
	EPHESUS – *NEJM*, 2003[30] 6,632 pts – EF <40% *3-14 d post-AMI*, NYHA 3-4 most on ACE-I (86%) *Eplerenone 25-50 mg/d vs. placebo*	15% RRR of death **NNT = 44** Effect seen mostly in sudden death 0.5% men had gynecomastia *Death in placebo arm lower than RALES (16.6% vs. 46%), EF higher (33% vs. 25%)*
Beta-Blockers	**CIBIS** – *Circulation*, 1994[19] 641 pts – EF <40%, NYHA 3 (95%)-4 (5%) on vasodilator and diuretic *Bisoprolol 1.25-5 mg/d vs. placebo*	All-cause mortality not stat significant 31% RRR of all CHF events **NNT = 6** 40% RR of NYHA improvement **NNT = 20** *55% RRR of death in pts with idiopathic dilated cardiomyopathy* **NNT = 9**
	CIBIS II – *Lancet*, 1999[20] 2,647 pts – EF <35%, NYHA 3-4, on diuretics, ACE-inhibitors *Bisoprolol 1.25-10 mg/d vs. placebo*	Stopped early due to mortality benefit 34% RRR of death **NNT = 18** 44% RRR of sudden death **NNT = 37**
	US Carvedilol Study – *NEJM*, 1996[21] 1,094 pts – EF <35%, NYHA 2-4 on diuretics and ACE-I *Carvedilol 6.25-25 mg bid vs. placebo*	Stopped early due to mortality benefit 65% RRR of death **NNT = 22** 27% RRR of CV admit **NNT = 18**

Drug	Trial and design	Results
Beta-Blockers (cont'd.)	**MERIT-HF** *Lancet*, 1999[23] 3,391 pts - NYHA 2-4 on diuretics, ACE-I *Metoprolol XL 12.5-200 mg/d vs. placebo*	Stopped early due to mortality benefit 33% RRR of death ***NNT = 26/pt y*** 49% RRR of death of CHF **NNT = 38** 41% RRR of sudden death **NNT = 71**
	BEST – *NEJM*, 2001[24] 2,708 pts – EF <35% NYHA 3-4 *Bucindolol 3-100 mg bid vs. placebo*	No overall mortality benefit 14% RRR of CV death **NNT = 25**
	COPERNICUS – NEJM, 2001[22] 2,289 pts – EF <25% NYHA 3-4 *Carvedilol 3.125-25 mg bid vs. placebo*	33% RRR of death **NNT = 18** 24% RRR of death or admit **NNT = 13**
	COMET – *Lancet*, 2003[25] 3,029 pts – EF <35%, NYHA II-IV, on diuretics + ACE-I unless not tolerated *Carvedilol 3.125-25 mg bid vs. metoprolol tartrate 5-50 mg bid*	17% RRR of death **NNT = 17** *1 y mortality in both arms higher than in MERIT-HF, CIBIS-II Used lower doses of metoprolol than MERIT-HF*
Nesiritide	**VMAC** – *JAMA*, 2002[33] 489 pts - acute decompensated CHF, NYHA 4 *Nesiritide 2 mcg/kg bolus then 0.01-0.03 mcg/kg/min vs NTG gtt vs placebo gtt*	At 3 hrs: PCWP -5.8 vs -3.8 vs -2 SOB improved vs placebo, not vs NTG At 24 hrs: PCWP -8.2 vs -6.3 NTG SOB same as with NTG Global clinical status not sig different

RR, relative risk; RRR, relative risk reduction; ARR, absolute risk reduction; NNT, number needed to treat = 1/ARR

REFERENCES

1. American Heart Association. *Heart Disease and Stroke Statistics: 2005 Update*. Dallas, TX: American Heart Association; 2005.
2. Koelling TM, Chen RS, Lubwama RN, et al. The expanding national burden of heart failure in the United States: The influence of heart failure in women. *Am Heart J.* 2004;147: 74–78.
3. Braunwald E, et al. *Braunwald's Heart Disease*, 7th ed., Saunders, 2004.

4. Stevenson LW, Perloff JK. The limited reliability of physical signs for estimating hemodynamics in chronic heart failure. *JAMA.* 1989;261:884–888.

5. Maisel AS, et al. Bedside B-Type natriuretic peptide in the emergency diagnosis of heart failure with reduced or preserved ejection fraction. Results from the Breathing Not Properly Multinational Study. *J Am Coll Cardiol.* 2003 Jun 4;41(11):2010–2017.

6. Maisel A. B-type natriuretic peptide levels: Diagnostic and prognostic in congestive heart failure: What's next? *Circulation.* 2002;105:2328.

7. Januzzi JL, van Kimmenade R, Lainchbury J, et al. NT-proBNP testing for diagnosis and short-term prognosis in acute destabilized heart failure: An international pooled analysis of 1256 patients: The International Collaborative of NT-proBNP Study. *Eur Heart J.* 2006;27:330.

8. Dormans T, et al. Diuretic efficacy of high-dose furosemide in severe heart failure: Bolus injection versus continuous infusion. *J Am Coll Cardiol.* 1996;23(2):376–382.

9. Rosenberg J, et al. Combination therapy with metolazone and loop diuretics in outpts with refractory heart failure: An observational study and review of the literature. *Cardiovasc Drugs Ther.* 2005;19:301–306.

10. Brater DC, et al. Bumetanide and furosemide in heart failure. *Kidney Int.* 1984;26:183–189.

11. Peter JV, et al. Effect of non-invasive positive pressure ventilation (NIPPV) on mortality in patients with acute cardiogenic pulmonary oedema: A metanalysis. *Lancet.* 2006;367:1155–1163.

12. The SOLVD Investigators. Effect of enalapril on mortality and the development of heart failure in asymptomatic patients with reduced left ventricular ejection fractions. *N Engl J Med.* 1992;327:685.

13. The CONSENSUS Trial Study Group. Effects of enalapril on mortality in severe congestive heart failure. Results of the Cooperative North Scandinavian Enalapril Survival Study (CONSENSUS). *N Engl J Med.* 1987;316:1429.

14. The SOLVD Investigators. Effect of enalapril on survival in patients with reduced left ventricular ejection fractions and congestive heart failure. *N Engl J Med.* 1991;325:293.

15. Granger CB, et al. Effects of candesartan in patients with chronic heart failure and reduced left-ventricular systolic function intolerant to angiotensin-converting-enzyme inhibitors: The CHARM-Alternative trial. *Lancet.* 2003;362:772.

16. Cohn JN, et al. Effect of vasodilator therapy on mortality in chronic congestive heart failure. Results of a Veterans Administration Cooperative Study. *N Engl J Med.* 1986;314:1547–1552.

17. Cohn JN, et al. A comparison of enalapril with hydralazine-isosorbide dinitrate in the treatment of chronic congestive heart failure. *N Engl J Med.* 1991;325:303–310.

18. Taylor AL, et al. Combination of isosorbide dinitrate and hydralazine in blacks with heart failure. *N Engl J Med.* 2004;351:2049–2057.
19. CIBIS Investigators. A randomized trial of beta-blockade in heart failure: The Cardiac Insufficiency Bisoprolol Study (CIBIS). *Circulation.* 1994;90:1765–1773.
20. CIBIS-II Investigators. The Cardiac Insufficiency Bisoprolol Study II (CIBIS-II): A randomized trial. *Lancet.* 1999;353:9–13.
21. Packer M, et al., for the US Carvedilol Heart Failure Study Group. The effect of carvedilol on morbidity and mortality in patients with chronic heart failure. *N Engl J Med.* 1996;334:1349–1355.
22. Packer M, et al., for the Carvedilol Prospective Randomized Cumulative Survival Study Group (COPERNICUS). Effect of carvedilol on survival in severe chronic heart failure. *N Engl J Med.* 2001;344:1651–1658.
23. Goldstein S, et al. Metoprolol controlled release/extended release in patients with severe heart failure. Analysis of the experience in the MERIT-HF study. *J Am Coll Cardiol.* 2001;38:932.
24. The BEST Trial Investigators. A trial of the beta-blocker bucindolol in patients with advanced chronic heart failure. *N Engl J Med.* 2001;344:1659–1667.
25. Poole-Wilson PA, et al. Comparison of carvedilol and metoprolol on clinical outcomes in patients with chronic heart failure in the Carvedilol Or Metoprolol European Trial (COMET): Randomised controlled trial. *Lancet.* 2003;362:7–13.
26. Bakris GL, et al. Metabolic effects of carvedilol vs. metoprolol in patients with type 2 diabetes mellitus and hypertension. *JAMA.* 2004;292:2227–2236.
27. Pitt B, Zannad F, Remme WJ, et al., for The Randomized Aldactone Evaluation Study (RALES) Investigators. The effect of spironolactone on morbidity and mortality in patients with severe heart failure. *N Engl J Med.* 1999;341:709.
28. Shah KB, et al. The adequacy of laboratory monitoring in patients treated with spironolactone for congestive heart failure. *J Am Coll Cardiol.* 2005;46:845–849.
29. Juurlink DN, et al. Rates of hyperkalemia after publication of the Randomized Aldactone Evaluation Study. *N Engl J Med.* 2004;351:543–551.
30. Neaton J. et al., for the Eplerenone Post-Acute Myocardial Infarction Heart Failure Efficacy and Survival Study (EPHESUS) Investigators. Eplerenone, a selective aldosterone blocker, in patients with left ventricular dysfunction after myocardial infarction. *N Engl J Med.* 2003;348:1309–1321.
31. The Digitalis Investigation Group. The effect of digoxin on mortality and morbidity in patients with heart failure. *N Engl J Med.* 1997;336:525.

32. Rathore SS, Curtis JP, Wang Y, et al. Association of serum digoxin concentration and outcomes in patients with heart failure. *JAMA*. 2003;289:871.

33. Publication Committee for the Vasodilation in the Management of Acute CHF (VMAC) Investigators. Intravenous nesiritide vs. nitroglycerin for treatment of decompensated congestive heart failure: A randomized controlled trial. *JAMA*. 2002;287: 1531–1540.

34. Colucci WS, Elkayam U, Horton DP, et al. Intravenous nesiritide, a natriuretic peptide, in the treatment of decompensated congestive heart failure. Nesiritide Study Group. *N Engl J Med*. 2000;343:246.

35. Burger AJ, Elkayam U, Neibaur MT, et al. Comparison of the occurrence of ventricular arrhythmias in patients with acutely decompensated congestive heart failure receiving dobutamine versus nesiritide therapy. *Am J Cardiol*. 2001;88:35.

36. Hunt SA, et al. ACC/AHA 2005 Guideline Update for the Diagnosis and Management of Chronic Heart Failure in the Adult: A report of the American College of Cardiology/American Heart Association Task Force on Practice Guidelines (Writing Committee to Update the 2001 Guidelines for the Evaluation and Management of Heart Failure). *Circulation*. 2005;112:e154.

37. Palazzuoli A, Carrera A, Calabria P, et al. Effects of carvedilol therapy on restrictive diastolic filling pattern in chronic heart failure. *Am Heart J*. 2004 Jan;147(1):E2.

38. Lonn E, et al. Effects of ramipril on left ventricular mass and function in cardiovascular patients with controlled blood pressure and with preserved left ventricular ejection fraction: A substudy of the Heart Outcomes Prevention Evaluation (HOPE) Trial. *J Am Coll Cardiol*. 2004 Jun 16;43(12):2200–2206.

39. Mottram PM, et al. Effect of aldosterone antagonism on myocardial dysfunction in hypertensive patients with diastolic heart failure. *Circulation*. 2004 Aug 3;110(5):558–565.

40. Pitt B, et al. Randomised trial of losartan versus captopril in patients over 65 with heart failure (Evaluation of Losartan in the Elderly Study, ELITE). *Lancet*. 1997;349:747–752.

41. Pitt B, et al. Effect of losartan compared with captopril on mortality in patients with symptomatic heart failure: Randomized trial—the Losartan Heart Failure Survival Study ELITE II. *Lancet*. 2000;355:1582–1587.

42. Pfeffer MA, et al. Effects of candesartan on mortality and morbidity in patients with chronic heart failure: The CHARM-Overall programme. *Lancet*. 2003;362:759–766.

43. McMurray JJV, et al. Effects of candesartan in patients with chronic heart failure and reduced left-ventricular systolic function taking

angiotension-converting enzyme inhibitors: The CHARM-Added trial. *Lancet*. 2003;362:767–771.

44. Yusuf S, et al. Effects of candesartan in patients with chronic heart failure and preserved left-ventricular ejection fraction: The CHARM-preserved trial. *Lancet*. 2003;362:777–781.

45. Cohn JN, Tognoni G, for the Valsartan Heart Failure Trial (ValHeFT) Investigators. A Randomized trial of the angiotensin-receptor blocker valsartan in chronic heart failure. *N Engl J Med.* 2001;345:1667–1675.

CHAPTER 10

Pulmonary Hypertension

FRANÇOIS HADDAD, RAMONA L. DOYLE, JULIANA C. LIU,
AND ROHAM T. ZAMANIAN

BACKGROUND

Pulmonary hypertension (PH) refers to a state in which pulmonary artery pressure is elevated. By expert consensus, PH is defined as a mean pulmonary arterial pressure (mPAP) greater than 25 mm Hg at rest or greater than 30 mm Hg with exercise as measured by right heart catheterization.[1] Pulmonary arterial hypertension (PAH) refers to disease states that localize to small pulmonary muscular arterioles. It is characterized as PH in the presence of (a) a pulmonary capillary wedge pressure (PCWP) <15 mm Hg, (b) pulmonary vascular resistance (PVR) >240 dynes/s/cm⁵ (3 Wood units), and (c) a transpulmonary gradient >10 mm Hg (mPAP-PCWP).[2]

GRADING THE SEVERITY OF PH

The severity of PH may be described in terms of pulmonary arterial pressure (Table 10-1), pulmonary vascular resistance or impedance, or pulmonary pathological vascular changes (Heath-Edwards classification [Table 10-2]). When assessing the severity of PH using levels of pulmonary arterial pressure, it is important to always consider cardiac output (CO). In fact, lower pulmonary arterial pressure may reflect a failing right ventricle and more advanced pulmonary vascular disease. Pulmonary vascular resistance (PVR) takes into account pulmonary pressure and flow and is measured as the difference between mean PAP and wedge pressure divided by cardiac output (PVR = (mPAP-PCWP)/CO). PVR is considered a better marker of pulmonary vascular disease. A normal value of PVR is 1 Wood unit or 80 dynes/s/cm⁵ while PVR values higher than

10 Wood units in PAH or value of PVR higher than 6 Wood units in left heart failure are considered severe. Pulmonary vascular histological changes of the media and intima have also been associated with the severity and reversibility of pulmonary arterial hypertension (PAH) associated with congenital heart disease or idiopathic PAH (Table 10-3).[3]

DEFINING PULMONARY VASCULAR REACTIVITY

Pulmonary vascular reactivity refers to the decrease in PAP in response to vasodilators. Several agents are of value in assessing acute vasoreactivity including oxygen, inhaled nitric oxide (usually 20 ppm), epoprostenol (Flolan), adenosine, or nitroprusside (especially in pre-heart transplant evaluations). Pulmonary vascular reactivity studies provide useful prognostic information and guide the choice of therapy in PAH, help predict the reparability of complex congenital heart disease, and help stratify the risk of acute right failure after heart transplantation. A positive vasodilator response in

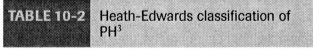

TABLE 10-1   Hemodynamic grading of PH

Severity	Mean PA (mm Hg)	Systolic PA (mm Hg)	Relative PA (mm Hg)
Mild	25–35	40–50	0.33–0.50
Moderate	35–50	50–80	0.50–0.66
Severe	>50	>80	>0.66

TABLE 10-2   Heath-Edwards classification of PH[3]

Pathologic grade	Pathology
Grade I	Hypertrophy of small muscular arteries and arterioles
Grade II	Grade I + intimal cell proliferation
Grade III	Obliterative arteriopathy
Grade IV	Plexiform lesion
Grade V	Complex plexiform, cavernous and angiomatous
Grade VI	Necrotizing arteritis

TABLE 10-3 Classification of pulmonary hypertension[1]

1. Pulmonary arterial hypertension (PAH)
    1.1. Idiopathic (IPAH)
    1.2. Familial (FPAH)
    1.3. Associated with (APAH):
    1.3.1. Collagen vascular disease
    1.3.2. Congenital systemic-to-pulmonary shunts
    1.3.3. Portal hypertension
    1.3.4. HIV infection
    1.3.5. Drugs and toxins
    1.3.6. Other (thyroid disorders, glycogen storage disease, Gaucher disease, hereditary hemorrhagic telangiectasia, hemoglobinopathies, myeloproliferative disorders, splenectomy)
    1.4. Associated with significant venous or capillary involvement
    1.4.1. Pulmonary veno-occlusive disease (PVOD)
    1.4.2. Pulmonary capillary hemangiomatosis (PCH)
    1.5. Persistent pulmonary hypertension of the newborn

2. Pulmonary hypertension with left heart disease
    2.1. Left-sided atrial or ventricular heart disease
    2.2. Left-sided valvular heart disease

3. Pulmonary hypertension associated with lung diseases and/or hypoxemia
    3.1. Chronic obstructive pulmonary disease
    3.2. Interstitial lung disease
    3.3. Sleep-disordered breathing
    3.4. Alveolar hypoventilation disorders
    3.5. Chronic exposure to high altitude
    3.6. Developmental abnormalities

4. Pulmonary hypertension due to chronic thrombotic and/or embolic disease
    4.1. Thromboembolic obstruction of proximal pulmonary arteries
    4.2. Thromboembolic obstruction of distal pulmonary arteries
    4.3. Nonthrombotic pulmonary embolism (tumor, parasites, foreign material)

5. Miscellaneous
Sarcoidosis, histiocytosis X, lymphangiomatosis, compression of pulmonary vessels (adenopathy, tumor, fibrosing mediastinitis)

PAH is defined as a reduction of mPAP by at least 10 mm Hg to a value of 40 mm Hg or less. Significant response is found in about 5% to 6% of PAH patients. These patients have a better response to calcium channel blockers.[2] A significant response in advanced heart disease undergoing a pretransplantation evaluation is defined by a decrease in PVR to a value of 3 Wood units or less.

WHO CLASSIFICATION OF PH

The World Health Organization (WHO) classifies patients with PH into five groups based on etiology and pathobiology. Pulmonary arterial hypertension (PAH) describes group 1 PAH; group 2 describes patients with pulmonary venous hypertension; group 3 refers to PH associated with lung disease and/or hypoxemia; group 4 describes PH associated with chronic thrombotic and/or embolic disease and group 5 refers to miscellaneous causes of PH.[1] This revised classification provides a useful framework for the diagnosis and management of PH patients. Modifications to this classification have been made at the latest WHO meeting in 2008. Formal publication of the classifications is still pending.

PATHOPHYSIOLOGY OF PH

Multiple molecular pathways have been implicated in the pathogenesis of PAH. These include nitric oxide, prostacyclin, endothelin-1, and serotonin pathways. A dysfunction in these pathways can lead to an imbalance between vasodilatation and vasoconstriction, and between apoptosis and proliferation, which leads to progressive vascular disease. In patients with pulmonary venous hypertension, PH can be explained by left ventricular diastolic failure, left-sided valvular heart disease, or pulmonary vein stenosis. In patients with lung disease, PH can be explained by hypoxemic vasoconstriction and/or by the loss of pulmonary vascular bed. In chronic thromboembolic PH (CTEPH), in situ thrombosis and/or failure of resolution of thromboemboli contribute to disease progression. The development of pulmonary hypertensive arteriopathy in unobstructive lung regions as well as in vessels distal to partially occluded proximal pulmonary arteries also contributes to the pathophysiology of CTEPH.

One of the most important consequences of PH is right ventricular (RV) failure. Survival in PH is closely related to RV failure. RV adaptation to disease depends on the time of onset of PH (congenital or acquired), setting (acute versus chronic), and specific cause of PH. Hypoxemia can be seen in PH as a result of right-to-left shunting through a patent foramen ovale or congenital defect, ventilation-perfusion mismatches, or decreased diffusion capacity. Hemoptysis, although rare, can be associated with significant morbidity and mortality. Hemoptysis may originate from a rupture of a bronchial artery or pulmonary trunk.

CLINICAL PRESENTATIONS

Most patients initially experience exertional dyspnea and fatigue, which reflects low cardiac output during exercise (low exercise reserve). As the PH progresses and RV failure develops, peripheral edema, exertional syncope, exertional chest pain, and passive liver congestion may occur. Less common symptoms of PH include cough, hemoptysis, and hoarseness (Ortner syndrome, which is due to compression of the left recurrent laryngeal nerve by a dilated main pulmonary artery). Other symptoms may also reflect the specific underlying cause.

Signs of RV failure are commonly found in patients with advanced PH; these include elevated jugular veins, distended liver, peripheral edema, and occasionally ascites. An increased intensity of the pulmonic component of the second heart sound is an initial physical finding in PH. Other signs include a right-sided S3 gallop, a holosystolic parasternal murmur of tricuspid regurgitation, and in more severe disease, a diastolic pulmonic regurgitation murmur. The right-sided murmurs and gallops are augmented with inspiration.[4]

LAB EXAMS AND IMAGING

A comprehensive workup is necessary in order to confirm the presence of PH, assess its severity and identify its cause.[1,2,5] *Echocardiography* is very helpful in estimating pulmonary artery pressure and assessing RV function. Signs of RV pressure overload may include D-shape left ventricle, tricuspid regurgitation, decreased systolic performance, and RV hypertrophy (>5 mm wall thickness). *Right heart catheterization (RHC)* is the most reliable method for measuring pulmonary arterial pressure, pulmonary vascular resistance, and pulmonary vascular reactivity. RHC is often obtained to confirm the diagnosis, assess pulmonary vascular reactivity, and evaluate the response to therapy. *Electrocardiography* may reveal signs of RV or right atrial dilatation, right bundle branch block, or arrhythmias. A *comprehensive laboratory workup* includes complete blood count, a comprehensive metabolic panel, B-type natriuretic peptide (BNP), troponins, collagen vascular disease workup, assessment for hypercoagulable states, hepatic serologies, and HIV screening. *Functional studies* such as 6-minute walk test or cardiopulmonary exercise test are important for the assessment of functional capacity and response to therapy. The diagnostic evaluation may also include a *pulmonary function test*, a *sleep study*, *chest x-ray*, *ventilation-perfusion scanning*, and/or *CT-angiography*. *Magnetic resonance imaging* is useful in studying RV function and in modeling pulmonary circulation.

HISTORY OF PH AND PROGNOSTIC FACTORS

Untreated idiopathic PAH (IPAH) is associated with a very poor prognosis with a 5-year survival rate of 34% according to the NIH registry.[6] PH is also recognized to be a bad prognostic factor in heart failure, valvular heart disease, pulmonary disease, and in systemic diseases such as scleroderma.[7] In PAH, factors associated with poor outcome include (a) low exercise capacity (NYHA: IV, 6 Minute Walk Distance <300 m [984 feet]); (b) markers of severe RV dysfunction including high right atrial pressure (RAP >15 mm Hg), low cardiac index, significant RV dysfunction, elevated BNP, and troponins; (c) rapid progression; (d) pericardial effusion; (e) poor response to prostacyclin therapy (persistence of NYHA III or IV); and (f) persistent supraventricular arrhythmias or sudden death.[2,8] In chronic thromboembolic PH, patients who are not considered suitable for pulmonary endarterectomy are considered at higher risk of mortality.[9]

MANAGEMENT OF PH

The management of pulmonary hypertension should be tailored to its cause, hemodynamic consequence (degree of RV failure), and vascular reactivity. Patients with significant PH should follow a low sodium diet (<2 grams of sodium), participate in graded physical activity, and avoid isometric activities such as weight lifting as well as medications that can exacerbate heart failure such as nonsteroidal anti-inflammatory medication. Pregnancy is also not advisable as maternal and fetal mortality can exceed 50%.

This revised WHO classification provides a useful framework for the management of PH patients. Patients with PAH (WHO class I) may benefit from prostanoid therapy (epoprostenol, treprostinil, iloprost), phosphodiesterase inhibitors (sildenafil), or an endothelin receptor antagonist (bosentan, ambrisentan). Anticoagulation with a goal INR between 1.5 to 2.5 is also recommended.[10] The minimal dose of diuretics is used to prevent fluid retention. The role of cardiac glycoside in pulmonary hypertension is controversial with only one study showing short-term hemodynamic benefits. The value of beta-blockade, angiotensin converting enzyme inhibitors, and spironolactone in chronic RV failure associated with PH has not been comprehensively studied. In patients presenting with acute decompensation, inhaled nitric oxide and vasopressor/inotropic support (usually with dobutamine 2 to 5 μg/kg/min) may be required (Figure 10-1 and Table 10-4). Atrial septostomy should only be considered a palliative procedure in refractory patients. Double-lung or heart-lung transplantation should be considered in selected patients.

In patients with pulmonary venous hypertension (WHO class II), optimization of left-sided heart failure and valvular disease management is the most important component of therapy. Small studies also suggest that sildenafil may be beneficial in selected patients with pulmonary hypertension.[11] In patients with PH secondary to lung disease and/or hypoxemia (WHO class III), primary therapy consists of oxygen therapy and ventilatory support (CPAP, BIPAP) as required. These patients usually do not benefit from treatment with pulmonary vasodilators. In patients with chronic thromboembolic disease (WHO class IV), therapy consists of anticoagulation and careful evaluation for candidacy for pulmonary endarterectomy.

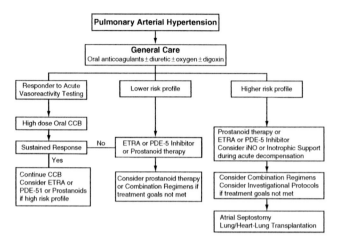

FIGURE 10-1 Algorithm for the management of PAH. Please refer to text for the definition of pulmonary reactivity and the description of higher risk patients. ETRA indicates endothelin receptor inhibitors; PDE-5, phosphodiesterase 5; CCB, calcium channel blockers. Prostanoid therapy includes intravenous epoprostenol, intravenous or subcutaneous treprostinil, and inhaled iloprost. (Adapted from McLaughlin VV, McGoon MD. Pulmonary arterial hypertension. *Circulation.* 2006 September 26;114[13]:1417–1431.)

TABLE 10-4	Characteristics of agents used in the treatment of PAH[1,2,4]			
Agent	Group Studied and Evidence	Effects	Dose and Characteristics	Significant Side Effects
Prostanoids				
Epoprostenol (Flolan)	PAH NYHA III–IV Randomized PC trials 12 weeks	1. ↑ 6MWT 2. Better HD 3. ↑ Survival (historical control)	Continuous IV Initiate: 1 ng/kg/min Usual: 30–40 ng/kg/min Half-life: 6 min	Jaw pain Hypotension May ↑ V/Q mismatch Catheter sepsis, thrombosis Rebound PH if D/C Thrombocytopenia

(continued)

TABLE 10-4 *(Continued)*

Agent	Group Studied and Evidence	Effects	Dose and Characteristics	Significant Side Effects
Treprostinil (Remodulin)	PAH NYHA III–IV Randomized PC trials 12 weeks	1. ↑ 6MWT 2. Better HD	SQ or IV Initiate: 1 ng/kg/min Usual: 40–60 ng/kg/min Half-life 3–4 h	Same as above except less rebound PH Possible ↑ incidence Gram – catheter sepsis Site pain with SQ form
Iloprost (Ventavis)	PAH NYHA III–IV Randomized PC trials 12 weeks	↑ in composite end point of improvement ↑ 6MWT	Inhalation (USA) 2.5-5 μg/inhalation 6 to 9 inhalations/d	Compliance difficult Variation PAP –
Endothelin receptor blockers				
Bosentan (nonselective)	PAH (Group 1) NYHA III–IV Randomized PC trials; 12 weeks	1. ↑ 6MWT 2. Better HD	125 mg po bid	Teratogenic ↑ Liver enzymes (10%)
Ambrisentan (selective)	Under review by FDA 06/07	1. ↑ 6MWT 2. Better HD	To be determined	Teratogenic ↑ Liver enzymes (3%)
Phospho-diesterase inhibitors				
Sildenafil	PAH NYHA II–III Randomized PC trials	1. ↑ 6MWT 2. Better HD	20 mg po tid	Hypotension Headache NAION (<1%) CI with nitrates
Calcium channel blockers	PAH-vasoreactive (<5%) Prospective trials	1. ↑ Survival in responders 2. Better HD 3. ↑ QL life	Higher doses Nifedipine ≈180 mg po daily	Hypotension Non-dihydropyridine → negative inotropy

Agent	Group Studied and Evidence	Effects	Dose and Characteristics	Significant Side Effects
Inhaled nitric oxide	PH Prospective studies	Better HD, oxygenation	20 ppm	Methemog-lobinemia Rebound PH

PH, pulmonary hypertension; PAH, pulmonary arterial hypertension; PC, placebo controlled; 6MWT, 6-minute walk test; HD, hemodynamic; NYHA, New York Heart Association Functional Class; NAION, nonarteritic anterior ischemic optic neuropathy

LANDMARK CLINICAL TRIALS

See Table 10-5.

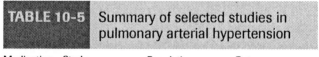

TABLE 10-5 Summary of selected studies in pulmonary arterial hypertension

Medication	Study	Population	n	Outcome
Prostacyclin (epoprostenol) continuous intravenous	The Primary PH Study Group[12] Randomized, 12 weeks	IPAH NYHA III–IV	81	1. ↑ 6MWT by 31 meters (60 meters comparative) in the prostacyclin group 2. HD improvement 3. Survival benefit
	Badesch et al.[13] Randomized, 12 weeks	Scleroderma spectrum of disease	113	1. ↑ 6MWT by 63 meters (99 meters comparative) in the prostacyclin group 2. HD improvement 3. No survival benefit
	Sitbon et al.[14] Observational long term	IPAH	178	Survival benefit compared to the historical control
	McLaughlin et al.[15] Observational long term	IPAH	162	Survival benefit compared to the historical control

(continued)

TABLE 10-5 *(Continued)*

Medication	Study	Population	n	Outcome
	Rosenweig et al.[16] Observational	CHD	20	Improvement in HD and exercise capacity (NYHA)
Treprostinil Subcutaneous intravenous	Subcutaneous Simonneau et al.[17] Randomized 12 weeks	PAH NYHA II–IV	470	1. Modest ↑ 6MWT by 16 meters 2. Dose-related improvement
	Intravenous Tapson et al.[18] Open-label prospective 12 weeks	PAH III–IV	16	1. ↑ 6MWT by 82 meters 2. Improvement in HD
	Intravenous Gomberg-Maitland et al.[19] Open-label Transition Study	PAH NYHA II–III	31	27 pts completed the transition and 4 were transitioned back to epoprostenol
Iloprost Inhaled (6-9 times daily)	Olschewski et al.[20] Randomized, 12 weeks	IPAH PAH-CTD PAH-stim. CTEPH (inoperable) NYHA III–IV	207	Improvement in composite end point of clinical improvement
Beraprost (not FDA approved)	Galie et al.[21] Randomized, 12 weeks	PAH NYHA II–III	130	1. ↑ 6MWT by 82 meters 2. No improvement in HD
	Barst et al.[22] Randomized 1 year	PAH NYHA II–III	116	No significant improvement in 6MWT at 9 and 12 meters
Bosentan (endothelin receptor blocker)	BREATHE-1[5] Randomized trial 12 weeks	IPAH PAH-CTD NYHA III–IV	213	1. ↑ 6MWT by 36 meters (44 meters comparative) 2. Improvement in time to clinical worsening
	McLaughlin et al.[23] Observational Long term	IPAH PAH-CTD NYHA III–IV	169	First-line bosentan ↑ survival compared to NIH historical control
	BREATHE-5[24] Randomized 16 weeks	CHD-Eisenmenger syndrome	54	1. ↑ 6MWT by 53 meters 2. HD improvement 3. No compromise peripheral oxygen saturation

Medication	Study	Population	n	Outcome
Sitaxsentan (ETA selective antagonist) (not FDA approved)	STRIDE-1[25] Randomized 12 weeks	PAH-IPAH,CTD,CHD NYHA II-IV	178	1. ↑ Maximum VO₂ 3.1%, sitaxsentan 300 mg, but unchanged 100 mg group 2. ↑ 6MWT
	SRIDE-2[26] Randomized 18 weeks	PAH-IPAH,CTD,CHD	247	1. ↑ 6MWT by 31 meters (100 mg dose)
Ambrisentan	Galie et al.[27] Randomized 12 weeks	PAH	64	1. ↑ 6MWT by 36 meters 2. HD improvement
Sildenafil	SUPER[28] Randomized 12 weeks	PAH-IPAH,CTD, repaired CHD	278	1. ↑ 6MWT by 45 meters placebo-corrected treatment effect 2. HD improvement

REFERENCES

1. Simonneau G, Galie N, Rubin LJ, et al. Clinical classification of pulmonary hypertension. *J Am Coll Cardiol.* 2004 June 16;43 (12 Suppl S):5S–12S.
2. McLaughlin VV, McGoon MD. Pulmonary arterial hypertension. *Circulation.* 2006 September 26;114(13):1417–1431.
3. Heath D, Edwards JE. The pathology of hypertensive pulmonary vascular disease; a description of six grades of structural changes in the pulmonary arteries with special reference to congenital cardiac septal defects. *Circulation.* 1958 October;18 (4 Part 1):533–547.
4. Rubin JR, Hopkins W. Overview of pulmonary hypertension. In: Rose BD, ed. *Up to Date.* Waltham, MA: 2007.
5. Rubin LJ, Badesch DB, Barst RJ, et al. Bosentan therapy for pulmonary arterial hypertension. *N Engl J Med.* 2002 March 21;346(12): 896–903.
6. D'Alonzo GE, Barst RJ, Ayres SM, et al. Survival in patients with primary pulmonary hypertension. Results from a national prospective registry. *Ann Intern Med.* 1991 September 1;115(5):343–349.
7. Haddad F, Doyle RL, Murphy DJ, et al. Right Ventricular Function in Cardiovascular Disease, Part II Pathophysiology, clinical importance and management of RV failure. *Circulation.* 2007. In press.
8. Tongers J, Schwerdtfeger B, Klein G, et al. Incidence and clinical relevance of supraventricular tachyarrhythmias in pulmonary hypertension. *Am Heart J.* 2007 January;153(1): 127–132.

9. Hoeper MM, Mayer E, Simonneau G, et al. Chronic thromboembolic pulmonary hypertension. *Circulation.* 2006 April 25;113(16):2011–2020.

10. McLaughlin VV, Rich S. Pulmonary hypertension. *Curr Probl Cardiol.* 2004 October;29(10):575–634.

11. Lewis GD, Lachmann J, Camuso J, et al. Sildenafil improves exercise hemodynamics and oxygen uptake in patients with systolic heart failure. *Circulation.* 2007 January 2;115(1):59–66.

12. Barst RJ, Rubin LJ, Long WA, et al. A comparison of continuous intravenous epoprostenol (prostacyclin) with conventional therapy for primary pulmonary hypertension. The Primary Pulmonary Hypertension Study Group. *N Engl J Med.* 1996 February 1;334(5):296–302.

13. Badesch DB, Tapson VF, McGoon MD, et al. Continuous intravenous epoprostenol for pulmonary hypertension due to the scleroderma spectrum of disease. A randomized, controlled trial. *Ann Intern Med.* 2000 March 21;132(6):425–434.

14. Sitbon O, Humbert M, Nunes H, et al. Long-term intravenous epoprostenol infusion in primary pulmonary hypertension: Prognostic factors and survival. *J Am Coll Cardiol.* 2002 August 21;40(4):780–788.

15. McLaughlin VV, Shillington A, Rich S. Survival in primary pulmonary hypertension: The impact of epoprostenol therapy. *Circulation.* 2002 September 17;106(12):1477–1482.

16. Rosenzweig EB, Kerstein D, Barst RJ. Long-term prostacyclin for pulmonary hypertension with associated congenital heart defects. *Circulation.* 1999 April 13;99(14):1858–1865.

17. Simonneau G, Barst RJ, Galie N, et al. Continuous subcutaneous infusion of treprostinil, a prostacyclin analogue, in patients with pulmonary arterial hypertension: A double-blind, randomized, placebo-controlled trial. *Am J Respir Crit Care Med.* 2002 March 15;165(6):800–804.

18. Tapson VF, Gomberg-Maitland M, McLaughlin VV, et al. Safety and efficacy of IV treprostinil for pulmonary arterial hypertension: A prospective, multicenter, open-label, 12-week trial. *Chest.* 2006 March;129(3):683–688.

19. Gomberg-Maitland M, Tapson VF, Benza RL, et al. Transition from intravenous epoprostenol to intravenous treprostinil in pulmonary hypertension. *Am J Respir Crit Care Med.* 2005 December 15;172(12):1586–1589.

20. Olschewski H, Simonneau G, Galie N, et al. Inhaled iloprost for severe pulmonary hypertension. *N Engl J Med.* 2002 August 1;347(5):322–329.

21. Galie N, Humbert M, Vachiery JL, et al. Effects of beraprost sodium, an oral prostacyclin analogue, in patients with pulmonary arterial hypertension: A randomized, double-blind, placebo-controlled trial. *J Am Coll Cardiol.* 2002 May 1;39(9):1496–1502.

22. Barst RJ, McGoon M, McLaughlin V, et al. Beraprost therapy for pulmonary arterial hypertension. *J Am Coll Cardiol.* 2003 June 18;41(12):2119–2125.
23. McLaughlin VV, Sitbon O, Badesch DB, et al. Survival with first-line bosentan in patients with primary pulmonary hypertension. *Eur Respir J.* 2005 February;25(2):244–249.
24. Galie N, Beghetti M, Gatzoulis MA, et al. Bosentan therapy in patients with Eisenmenger syndrome: A multicenter, double-blind, randomized, placebo-controlled study. *Circulation.* 2006 July 4;114(1):48–54.
25. Barst RJ, Langleben D, Frost A, et al. Sitaxsentan therapy for pulmonary arterial hypertension. *Am J Respir Crit Care Med.* 2004 February 15;169(4):441–447.
26. Barst RJ, Langleben D, Badesch D, et al. Treatment of pulmonary arterial hypertension with the selective endothelin-A receptor antagonist sitaxsentan. *J Am Coll Cardiol.* 2006 May 16;47(10):2049–2056.
27. Galie N, Badesch D, Oudiz R, et al. Ambrisentan therapy for pulmonary arterial hypertension. *J Am Coll Cardiol.* 2005 August 2;46(3):529–535.
28. Galie N, Ghofrani HA, Torbicki A, et al. Sildenafil citrate therapy for pulmonary arterial hypertension. *N Engl J Med.* 2005 November 17;353(20):2148–2157.

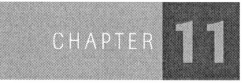

CHAPTER 11

Transplant Medicine

MICHAEL PHAM

BACKGROUND

The first human heart transplant was performed in South Africa in 1967, followed by the first U.S. procedure in 1968 by Dr. Norman Shumway at Stanford University. Over 4,000 heart transplants are performed worldwide each year; the number of procedures is currently limited by the availability of organ donors. Survival rates are 81%, 74%, 68%, and 50% at 1, 3, 5, and 10 years.[1]

INDICATIONS FOR TRANSPLANTATION

- Systolic heart failure with severe functional limitation and/or refractory symptoms despite maximal medical therapy
  - Left ventricular ejection fraction (LVEF) usually <35%, but a low LVEF is not an adequate indication for transplantation
  - NYHA Functional Class III-IV
  - Maximum oxygen uptake (VO$_2$ max) of $\leq$12 to 14 cc/kg/min on exercise testing
- Cardiogenic shock not expected to recover
  - Acute myocardial infarction
  - Myocarditis
- Ischemic heart disease with intractable angina
  - Not amenable to surgical or percutaneous revascularization
  - Refractory to maximal medical therapy
- Intractable ventricular arrhythmias, uncontrolled with antiarrhythmic medications, ICD therapy, and/or ablation
- Severe symptomatic hypertrophic or restrictive cardiomyopathy
- Congenital heart disease
- Cardiac tumors with low likelihood of metastasis

CONTRAINDICATIONS

* Irreversible severe pulmonary arterial hypertension: Considered an *absolute* contraindication by most programs

  ○ Pulmonary vascular resistance (PVR) >4 to 5 Wood units
  ○ Pulmonary vascular resistance index (PVRI) >6
  ○ Transpulmonary gradient (mean PA − PCWP) >16 to 20 mm Hg
  ○ PA systolic pressure >50 to 60 mm Hg or >50% of systemic pressures

* Advanced age: Many programs are moving away from "absolute" age limits and considering rehabilitation potential, end-organ function, and presence of comorbid conditions when evaluating older patients. Some programs still have an age cutoff between 65 and 70 years of age.
* Active systemic infection: Patients can typically be listed after the infection has been identified and adequately treated (i.e., absence of fever, leukocytosis, and bacteremia).
* Active malignancy or recent malignancy with high risk of recurrence. Exceptions include nonmelanoma skin cancers, primary cardiac tumors restricted to the heart, and low-grade prostate cancers. Consultation with an oncologist is recommended.
* Diabetes mellitus with either poor glycemic control (variable definitions, but usually HbA1c >7.5) or end-organ damage (neuropathy, nephropathy, and proliferative retinopathy)
* Marked obesity (body mass index [BMI] >30 kg/m^2 or >140% of ideal body weight). Most programs will have variable cutoffs for BMI.
* Severe peripheral arterial disease not amenable to revascularization
* Systemic process with high probability of recurrence in the transplanted heart

  ○ Amyloidosis
  ○ Sarcoidosis
  ○ Hemochromatosis

* Irreversible severe renal, hepatic, or pulmonary disease. Occasional combined heart/kidney, heart/lung, or heart/liver transplants are done at selected centers.
* Recent or unresolved pulmonary infarction due to the high probability of progression into pulmonary abscesses after initiating immunosuppression
* Psychosocial factors that may impact on patient's ability to receive posttransplant care

  ○ History of poor compliance with medications or follow-up appointments
  ○ Lack of adequate support system
  ○ Uncontrolled psychiatric illness
  ○ Active or recent substance abuse (alcohol, tobacco, or illicit drugs)

PRETRANSPLANT EVALUATION

History

* Does patient meet indications for transplantation?
* Has adequate medical, device, and/or surgical therapy been attempted?
* Does patient have significant contra-indications to transplantation?

Psychosocial Evaluation

* Assess patient's understanding of transplant procedure and willingness to undergo lifelong immunosuppression and follow-up
* Assess adequacy of social support system
* Assess for uncontrolled psychiatric illness or active/recent substance abuse that may impact posttransplant care.

Lab Exams and Imaging

* Blood tests: Complete blood count, electrolytes, renal and hepatic function, ABO typing; human leukocyte antigens (HLA) antibody screen against panel of common antigens (PRA); hepatitis, syphilis, and HIV serologies
* Chest x-ray
* Electrocardiogram
* Echocardiogram
* Coronary angiography (or review most recent study) if known coronary artery disease (CAD) or if patient has risk factors for CAD
* Right heart catheterization to document pulmonary artery pressures. Pharmacologic intervention with vasodilators (intravenous nitride or inhaled nitric oxide) may be used to document reversibility of pulmonary hypertension.
* Pulmonary function testing
* Carotid ultrasound and lower extremity ABIs
* Age and sex-appropriate cancer screening (PAP smear, mammogram, colonoscopy, prostate-specific antigen (PSA) with DRE)

Most candidacy determinations are made after review of patient's history and workup by a multidisciplinary Transplant Selection Committee comprising cardiologists, surgeons, social workers, and/or psychologists.

ORGAN MATCHING AND PRIORITIZATION

* Recipient waiting list maintained by United Network of Organ Sharing (UNOS)
* Recipients and donors are matched by blood type, weight, priority status (Table 11-1), and time accrued on waiting list.
* Prospective HLA matching between donor and recipient is typically *not* performed unless a recipient has high levels of preformed antibodies (PRA >20%).

TABLE 11-1	UNOS prioritization of heart transplant recipients

Status	Criteria	Location
1A	Mechanical circulatory support, or • ventricular assist device (VAD) (first 30 days) or total artificial heart (TAH) • intra-aortic balloon pump (IABP) or extracorporeal membrane oxygenation (ECMO) Mechanical ventilation Inotropic requirement *with* HD monitoring • 1 high-dose (Dob ≥7.5, mcg/kg/min milrinone ≥0.5 mcg/kg/min) • 2 inotropes (IV vasodilators do *not* count) Exceptional provision (life expectancy <14 d)	Transplant center
1B	• 1 inotrope, or • VAD after 30 days	Hospital or outpatient
2	Not meeting criteria for 1A or 1B listing (stable)	
7	On hold (infection, insurance, clearance too well)	

- Waiting times range from days to years and are dependent upon priority status (shortest for 1A, longest for 2), blood type (longest for blood group O), weight (longer for large recipients), and geographic location.

SURGICAL TECHNIQUE

- Most donor hearts are implanted in the orthotopic position (i.e., in the same position as the explanted heart).
- The original technique involved anastomosis of the donor heart at the level of the atria (*biatrial technique*), leaving a cuff of donor atria. In recent years, the biatrial technique has been modified to make the anastomoses at the level of the superior and inferior vena cavae and pulmonary veins (*bicaval technique*). This results in less A-V valve regurgitation, decreased incidence of atrial arrhythmias, and decreased incidence of donor sinus node dysfunction and heart block requiring permanent pacemaker implantation.
- Ischemic times of 3 to 4 hours are preferred.

PHYSIOLOGY OF TRANSPLANTED HEART

● The transplanted heart is initially completely denervated. Cardiac denervation has several important clinical implications:

  ○ Patients exhibit a faster resting heart rate (usually between 95 to 110 bpm)
  ○ Many patients will not experience angina. Typical presentations of ischemia include congestive heart failure, myocardial infarction, or sudden death.
  ○ Drugs that act through the autonomic nervous system (e.g., atropine) will have little to no effect on a transplanted heart.

IMMUNOSUPPRESSION

General Principles

● The risk of rejection is highest immediately after transplantation and decreases over time. Most rejection episodes occur during the first year; therefore, immunosuppression is highest during this time.
● The goal of immunosuppression is to use the lowest doses of drugs to prevent rejection while minimizing toxicities (particularly renal insufficiency) and immunosuppression-related complications (infection and cancer).

Induction Therapy

● Currently, induction is used by 50% of transplant centers to provide a period of intense immunosuppression in the early (first 6 months) posttransplant period, when the risk of rejection is highest.
● Advantages: Decreases the incidence of rejection during the first 6 months, allows delayed initiation of nephrotoxic immunosuppressive drugs in patients with compromised renal function after surgery
● Disadvantages: May simply be shifting rejection to the late period (6–12 months) after transplantation; may increase the risk of infection and malignancy
● Agents used for induction include

  ○ Cytolytic agents are antibodies that result in near complete depletion of T-lymphocytes (OKT3, Thymoglobulin)
  ○ Interleukin-2 receptor antagonists are antibodies that inhibit IL-2 mediated proliferation of activated T-lymphocytes (daclizumab, basiliximab).

Maintenance Immunosuppression

Most maintenance protocols employ a two- to three-drug regimen with no more than one agent from each class to avoid overlapping toxicities (see Table 11-2). The dosing, target drug levels, and side effect profile of each agent is shown in Table 11-3.

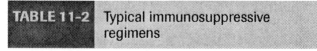

TABLE 11-2   Typical immunosuppressive regimens

Era	Pre-1980s	Typical	CAV	Renal sparing
Calcineurin inhibitor		Cyclosporine or tacrolimus	Cyclosporine or tacrolimus	
Antiproliferative agent	Imuran	Mycophenolate mofetil		Mycophenolate mofetil
mTOR inhibitor			Sirolimus	Sirolimus
Corticosteroids	Prednisone (lifelong)	Prednisone (first 6–12 mo)		

TABLE 11-3   Immunosuppressive agents used in heart transplantation

Drug	Dosing	Target Levels	Major Toxicities
Calcineurin inhibitors			
Cyclosporine	4–8 mg/kg/d in two divided doses, titrated to keep target 12-h trough levels	0–6 Months: 250–350 ng/mL 6–12 Months: 200–250 ng/mL >12 Months: 100–200 ng/mL	Renal insufficiency Hypertension Dyslipidemia Hypokalemia and hypomagnesemia Hyperuricemia Neurotoxicity (encephalopathy, seizures, tremors, neuropathy, posterior reversible encephalopathy syndrome [PRES]) Gingival hyperplasia Hirsutism
Tacrolimus	0.05-0.1 mg/kg/d in two divided doses, titrated to keep target 12-h trough levels	0–6 Months: 10–14 ng/mL 6–12 Months: 7–10 ng/mL >12 Months: 5–10 ng/mL	Renal dysfunction Hypertension Hyperglycemia and diabetes mellitus Dyslipidemia Hyperkalemia Hypomagnesemia Neurotoxicity (tremors, headaches, PRES)

Drug	Dosing	Target Levels	Major Toxicities
Antiproliferative agents			
Azathioprine	1.5–3.0 mg/kg/d, titrated to keep WBC ~3,000	None	Bone marrow suppression Hepatitis (rare) Pancreatitis Malignancy
Mycophenolate mofetil	1,000–3,000 mg/d in two divided doses	Mycophenolic acid (MPA): 2.5–4.5 μg/mL	Gastrointestinal disturbances (nausea, diarrhea) Leukopenia
mTOR inhibitors			
Sirolimus	1-3 mg/d, titrated to keep therapeutic 24-h trough levels	5-10 ng/mL	Oral ulcerations Hypercholesterolemia and hypertriglyceridemia Poor wound healing Lower extremity edema Pneumonitis Leukopenia, anemia, and thrombocytopenia Potentiation of CNI nephrotoxicity
Corticosteroids			
Prednisone	1 mg/kg/d in two divided doses, tapered to 0.05 mg/kg/d by 6–12 mo	None	Weight gain Hypertension Hyperlipidemia Osteopenia Hyperglycemia Poor wound healing Salt and water retention Proximal myopathy Cataracts Peptic ulcer disease Growth retardation

- *Calcineurin inhibitors*: Block calcineurin-dependent signal transduction, thus inhibiting IL-2 production and preventing both T- and B-cell differentiation and proliferation. They are the cornerstone of immunosuppression in heart transplantation.
  - Cyclosporine (Sandimmune, Neoral, Gengraf) was introduced in the 1980s and led to a dramatic decrease in acute rejection and subsequent increase in life expectancy after heart transplantation.
  - Tacrolimus (Prograf) is similar in efficacy to cyclosporine but has a more favorable metabolic profile (less hypertension and dyslipidemia)

and lacks cyclosporin-specific side effects such as hirsutism and gingival hyperplasia.[2,3] In the kidney transplant literature, use of tacrolimus is associated with a higher incidence of posttransplant diabetes compared to cyclosporine, and a similar trend has been noted in heart transplant patients.

- *Antiproliferative agents*: Block purine synthesis and inhibit proliferation of both T- and B-lymphocytes
  - Mycophenolate mofetil (CellCept) has replaced the older agent, azathioprine (Imuran) as the preferred antiproliferative agent in recent years.[4]
- *Mammalian Target of Rapamycin (mTOR) inhibitors*[5,6] are a newer class of agents that block proliferation of T-cells, B-cells, and vascular smooth muscle cells by causing cell cycle arrest at the G1 to S phase. They are used in patients with cardiac allograft vasculopathy (CAV) due to their antiproliferative effects on vascular smooth muscle cells and in patients with renal insufficiency because they have no intrinsic nephrotoxic effects.
  - Sirolimus (Rapamune)
  - Everolimus (Certican) is used in Europe and undergoing Phase III clinical trials in the United States.
- Glucocorticoids are nonspecific agents that are typically used in high doses in the early posttransplant period and then tapered to low doses or discontinued altogether after the first 6 to 12 months.

DRUG INTERACTIONS

Many drugs can alter the metabolism of the immunosuppressive agents, and vice versa (Table 11-4).[7]

REJECTION

Even with modern immunosuppressive regimens, acute rejection is still experienced by 30% to 50% of patients during the first year after transplantation.

Types of Rejection

1. Hyperacute rejection: Very rare and may occur immediately after transplantation in the setting of high levels of preformed antibodies to the ABO blood group (in cases of incompatibility) or to major histocompatibility antigens in the donor.
2. Acute cellular rejection (ACR): The most common form of rejection and mediated by T-lymphocytes. It is detected by identifying lymphocytic infiltration, inflammation, and myocyte damage on heart

TABLE 11-4   Important drug interactions

Increase levels of cyclosporine, tacrolimus, and sirolimus

Calcium channel blockers	Diltiazem Nifedipine Nicardipine Verapamil
Antifungal drugs	Itraconazole Fluconazole Ketoconazole Voriconazole Posaconazole
Macrolide antibiotics	All
Fluoroquinolone antibiotics	Ciprofloxacin
HIV-protease inhibitors	All
Antiarrhythmic agents	Amiodarone
Gastrointestinal agents	Metoclopramide
Miscellaneous	Grapefruit juice

Decrease levels of cyclosporine, tacrolimus, and sirolimus

Antitubercular drugs	Rifampin
Antiseizure drugs	Phenytoin Phenobarbital
Gastrointestinal drugs	Octreotide
Miscellaneous	Saint-John's-wort

Drugs with synergistic nephrotoxicity when used with cyclosporine or tacrolimus

Aminoglycoside antibiotics Amphotericin B Colchicine Nonsteroidal anti-inflammatory agents (NSAIDs)	

Drugs whose concentrations are increased when used with with cyclosporine or tacrolimus

Lovastatin Simvastatin Atorvastatin Ezetimibe	

biopsy samples. ACR is graded according to a standardized classification system developed by the International Society of Heart and Lung Transplantation (ISHLT). (Table 11-5).[8]

3. Acute antibody mediated rejection (AMR) is mediated by B-lymphocytes and characterized by immunoglobulin deposition on the cardiac allograft microvasculature, causing complement activation, myocardial injury, and eventual graft dysfunction. Compared to ACR, AMR is more likely to cause hemodynamic instability and is associated with a worse prognosis. It is detected by a combination of histologic evidence of capillary injury, positive immunohistochemistry staining for C4d (a complement split product), or immunofluorescence staining for immunoglobulin deposition on heart biopsy specimens, clinical evidence of graft dysfunction, and by measuring HLA antibodies in the circulation that are directed against known donor antigens.

TABLE 11-5 Acute rejection grading and treatment

Acute cellular rejection (ACR)

Severity	Old (1990) ISHLT Grade	Revised (2004) ISHLT Grade	Pathologic Features	Treatment
No rejection	0	0R	Normal myocardium	None
Mild	1A, 1B, 2	1R	Interstitial and/or perivascular mononuclear cell infiltrate with up to one focus of myocyte damage	None; optimize maintenance immuno-suppression
Moderate	3A	2R	Two or more foci of mononuclear cell infiltrate with associated myocyte damage	*No hemodynamic compromise* Pulse steroids (methylpredniso-lone 500–1,000 mg IV daily × 3 days) *Hemodynamic compromise* Pulse steroids *and/or* cytolytic antibody therapy (OKT3, ATGAM, or Thymoglobulin)

Severe	3B, 4	3R	Diffuse mononuclear and/or mixed inflammatory cell infiltrates with multiple foci of myocyte damage, with or without edema, hemorrhage, or vasculitis	Pulse steroids *and/or* cytolytic antibody therapy (OKT3, rATG)

Antibody-mediated rejection (AMR)

Absent or present		AMR 0 (absent) or 1 (present)	Absence of cellular infiltrate; prominent endothelial cells lining microvasculature; presence of intravascular histiocytes; interstitial edema; positive immunofluorescence or immunoperoxidase staining (CD68, C4d)	Pulse steroids Plasmapheresis Photopheresis IV immunoglobulin Cytolytic antibody therapy (OKT3, rATG) Rituximab

Treatment

* Rejection episodes are treated by augmentation of immunosuppression. The specific treatment depends upon the type of rejection, histologic severity of rejection episode, and presence of graft dysfunction or hemodynamic compromise (defined as a decrease in left ventricular systolic function, decrease in cardiac output, or signs of hypoperfusion) (Table 11-5).
* Any rejection episode should prompt an investigation for precipitating causes (CMV infection, noncompliance, drug interactions resulting in subtherapeutic immunosuppressive drug levels).
* A biopsy should be repeated 2 weeks after completion of treatment to document resolution of a rejection episode.
* Recurrent or recalcitrant rejection can be treated with total lymphoid irradiation.

CARDIAC ALLOGRAFT VASCULOPATHY (CAV)

CAV is a major cause of late graft failure and death in heart transplant patients. It is noted angiographically in 10% of patients by the first postoperative year and in 30% to 50% of patients by the fifth posttransplant year.

CAV Pathogenesis

The pathogenesis of CAV is not completely understood, but it is thought to involve both immune and nonimmune mechanisms. It manifests as diffuse coronary intimal thickening with tapering or pruning of distal vessels. However, focal stenoses can also be present.

CAV Diagnosis

CAV is detected on the basis of surveillance coronary angiography, although the disease can be difficult to detect due to its diffuse nature. Some centers use intravascular ultrasound (IVUS) as a more sensitive tool for early CAV detection. Dobutamine stress echocardiography (DSE) provides a reasonable alternative to yearly coronary angiography when used to screen for CAV. In this setting, a normal DSE predicts a low risk of major adverse cardiac events over the next year.[9]

CAV Treatment

The mTOR inhibitors (sirolimus and everolimus) have been shown to slow progression of the disease.[5,6] PCI with stenting can be effective for focal lesions.[10] Outcomes following coronary artery bypass graft (CABG) for CAV have been poor.[11] The most definitive form of treatment is retransplantation and is typically reserved for patients with severe, symptomatic CAV and graft failure.[12]

EVALUATION AND MANAGEMENT OF A HEART TRANSPLANT PATIENT WITH HEART FAILURE

- New onset of heart failure signs or symptoms in a transplant patient constitutes a *medical emergency.*
- Heart failure can be caused by both *systolic* and *diastolic* dysfunction. The echocardiogram can be useful to document a reduction in LV systolic function, but a normal LVEF does not exclude the possibility of graft dysfunction.
- The etiology of heart failure varies according to time posttransplant
  - *Early period (years 1-2)*: Acute rejection >> CAV resulting in silent ischemia or infarction
  - *Late period (years 2 and beyond)*: CAV >> acute rejection

Workup includes an echocardiogram, electrocardiogram, right heart catheterization, heart biopsy (if rejection is suspected), and coronary angiography (if CAV is suspected).

- The patient's transplant team should be contacted immediately, and prompt transfer to a transplant center should be arranged if the patient presents to an outside hospital.
- In the early period (years 1–2 after transplantation), consider administration of high-dose steroids (methylprednisolone 1 gm IV) to pre-emptively treat for possible rejection until additional testing can be performed.

OPPORTUNISTIC INFECTIONS

Infections are a major cause of death during the first year and remain a threat throughout the life of a chronically immunosuppressed patient. Effective therapy requires an aggressive approach to obtaining specific microbiological diagnosis (i.e., bronchoscopy with bronchoalveolar lavage for pneumonias, fine needle aspiration for pulmonary nodules, detection of CMV viremia via quantitative PCR of the serum).

* Bacterial pathogens are more likely to cause disease in the first month and are typically associated with indwelling catheters and surgical wounds.
* Viral pathogens include cytomegalovirus (CMV) and herpes simplex virus (HSV).
* Fungal pathogens include *Aspergillus*, *Candida*, and *Pneumocystis*.
* Atypical pathogens include *Mycobacterium*, *Nocardia*, and *Toxoplasma*.

REFERENCES

1. Taylor DO, Edwards LB, Boucek MM, et al. Registry of the International Society for Heart and Lung Transplantation: Twenty-third official adult heart transplantation report—2006. *J Heart Lung Transplant.* Aug 2006;25(8):869–879.
2. Taylor DO, Barr ML, Radovancevic B, et al. A randomized, multicenter comparison of tacrolimus and cyclosporine immunosuppressive regimens in cardiac transplantation: Decreased hyperlipidemia and hypertension with tacrolimus. *J Heart Lung Transplant.* Apr 1999;18(4):336–345.
3. Reichart B, Meiser B, Vigano M, et al. European Multicenter Tacrolimus (FK506) Heart Pilot Study: One-year results—European Tacrolimus Multicenter Heart Study Group. *J Heart Lung Transplant.* Aug 1998;17(8):775–781.
4. Kobashigawa J, Miller L, Renlund D, et al. A randomized active-controlled trial of mycophenolate mofetil in heart transplant recipients. Mycophenolate Mofetil Investigators. *Transplantation.* Aug 27 1998;66(4):507–515.
5. Keogh A, Richardson M, Ruygrok P, et al. Sirolimus in de novo heart transplant recipients reduces acute rejection and prevents coronary artery disease at 2 years: A randomized clinical trial. *Circulation.* Oct 26 2004;110(17):2694–2700.
6. Eisen HJ, Tuzcu EM, Dorent R, et al. Everolimus for the prevention of allograft rejection and vasculopathy in cardiac-transplant recipients. *N Engl J Med.* Aug 28 2003;349(9):847–858.
7. Page RL II, Miller GG, Lindenfeld J. Drug therapy in the heart transplant recipient: Part IV: Drug-drug interactions. *Circulation.* Jan 18 2005;111(2):230–239.

8. Stewart S, Winters GL, Fishbein MC, et al. Revision of the 1990 working formulation for the standardization of nomenclature in the diagnosis of heart rejection. *J Heart Lung Transplant.* Nov 2005; 24(11):1710–1720.

9. Spes CH, Klauss V, Mudra H, et al. Diagnostic and prognostic value of serial dobutamine stress echocardiography for noninvasive assessment of cardiac allograft vasculopathy: A comparison with coronary angiography and intravascular ultrasound. *Circulation.* Aug 3 1999;100(5):509–515.

10. Bader FM, Kfoury AG, Gilbert EM, et al. Percutaneous coronary interventions with stents in cardiac transplant recipients. *J Heart Lung Transplant.* Mar 2006;25(3):298–301.

11. Halle AA III, DiSciascio G, Massin EK, et al. Coronary angioplasty, atherectomy and bypass surgery in cardiac transplant recipients. *J Am Coll Cardiol.* Jul 1995;26(1):120–128.

12. Topkara VK, Dang NC, John R, et al. A decade experience of cardiac retransplantation in adult recipients. *J Heart Lung Transplant.* Nov 2005;24(11):1745–1750.

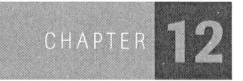

CHAPTER 12

Valvular Diseases

SHRIRAM NALLAMSHETTY AND STANLEY G. ROCKSON

AORTIC STENOSIS

Background
* The normal aortic valve orifice area (AVA) is 3 to 4 cm^2; clinically significant gradients occur when AVA is reduced by one half, and symptoms usually arise when AVA is one fourth of normal size.
* Grading severity is based on valve area, gradients, and aortic jet velocity.[1,2] (See Table 12-1.)
* Gradients are less predictive (a mean gradient > 50 mm Hg has >90% positive predictive value for severe AS, but there is no clear cutoff for a good negative predictive value[3]).

Etiology
* Most common etiologies: Congenital, rheumatic, and calcific (degenerative) (See Table 12-2.)
* Under 70 years: >50% congenital; over 70 years: ~ 50% degenerative[4]

Pathophysiology
* Pressure gradient between the left ventricle (LV) and aorta (increased afterload)
* Initially, cardiac output is maintained through compensatory mechanisms of left ventricular hypertrophy (LVH), increased preload, and increased myocardial contractility.
* If preload reserve is exceeded or if LV function declines, cardiac output fails to increase (fixed cardiac output).

History
* Cardinal manifestations: Classic triad of angina, exertional syncope, and congestive heart failure (CHF).
* Angina is due to increased myocardial demand/decreased coronary flow reserve.[6]
* Syncope can be due to exercise-related vasodilation in the setting of fixed cardiac output,[7] as well as a vasodepressor response.[8]

179

TABLE 12-1	Grading of severity of AS	
Severity of AS	AVA	Velocity
Mild	$>1.5\,cm^2$	2.6–3.0 m/s
Moderate	$1.0–1.5\,cm^2$	3.0–4.0 m/s
Severe	$<1.0\,cm^2$	$>4.0\,m/s$

TABLE 12-2	Etiology of AS
Etiology	Notes
Congenital	
1. Congenital aortic stenosis	Can occur with unicuspid, bicuspid, tricuspid valve
2. Congenital bicuspid valve	Commonly associated with aortic coarctation, dissection, or aneurysm. Onset of symptoms in third to fifth decade
Acquired	
1. Degenerative calcification	Onset of symptoms in seventh to eighth decade. Higher incidence of risk factors for coronary artery disease (CAD)
2. Rheumatic heart disease	Adhesions and fusion of commissures and cusps
3. Rare causes	Infectious vegetations, Paget disease, SLE, RA, Postradiation (typically occurs 11.5–16.5 years after radiation[5])

- CHF results from diastolic dysfunction, systolic dysfunction, or both.
- Sudden cardiac death occurs in a minority of patients (less than 1% of asymptomatic patients; higher rates among symptomatic patients).[2,9,10]

Natural History
- Progression of AS is poorly understood; the latent phase is prolonged.
- Rate of progression
  - Mild AS to severe AS: 8% in 10 years, 22% in 20 years, and 38% in 25 years[11]
  - Decrease in valve area of 0.1 to $0.3\,cm^2$/year and increase in peak pressure gradient of 10 to 15 mm Hg/year[12–14]
  - Faster progression in calcific AS than in congenital malformations[15]
- The onset of symptoms marks an important transition with a marked decline in survival (50% survival over 2, 3, and 5 years for patients with CHF, syncope, and exertional angina, respectively).[16]
- Presence of symptoms may be difficult to gauge, especially in sedentary/elderly individuals.

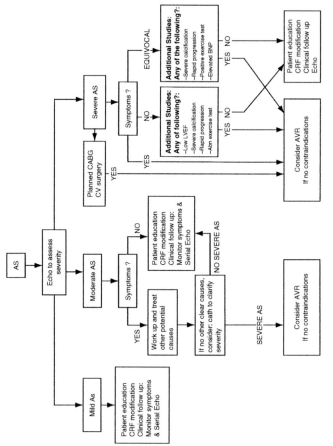

FIGURE 12-1 Management algorithm: aortic stenosis.

181

Physical Exam

- Systolic ejection murmur is heard best in the aortic area/apex radiating to neck and right clavicle.
- Gallavardin phenomenon (disappearance of the murmur over the sternum and reappearance over the apex, mimicking mitral regurgitation (MR))
- Intensity of murmur does not accurately reflect severity of stenosis.
- Later peaking murmur is associated with worsening severity of stenosis.
- S_2 is absent, single, paradoxically split in severe AS.
- *Pulsus parvus et tardus* (slow rising arterial pulse with reduced peak) in severe AS

Lab Exams and Imaging

- Brain natriuretic peptide (BNP) may be useful in differentiating symptomatic from asymptomatic patients (BNP >66 pg/mL has predictive accuracy of 84% for symptomatic AS).[17,18]
- Chest x-ray can show dilated proximal ascending aorta (poststenotic dilatation) and calcification of cusps on lateral films.
- Electrocardiogram
  - Usually normal sinus rhythms (NSR), but AF is common in elderly AS patients
  - Complete heart block may occur in calcific AS
  - Left atrial enlargement present in 80% of patients
  - LVH with secondary ST-T changes
- Echo
  - Useful for diagnosis, determining severity (AVA, velocity, gradient; see Table 12-1)
  - AVA is determined using the continuity equation (conservation of mass).
  - Peak pressure gradient is determined using Continuous Wave (CW) Doppler.
  - Accuracy compared to cardiac catheterization:[19] Valve area is within ±0.3 cm;[2] Peak gradient is within ±10 mm Hg; Gradients usually higher than cath due to pressure recovery[20]
- Recommendations for serial studies (in the absence of symptoms)[1]
- Mild: Every 5 years
- Moderate: Every 2 years
- Severe: Every 6 months to 1 year

Provocative Testing

EXERCISE TESTING

- Contraindicated in symptomatic patients
- Should be considered in patients severe AS, with unclear symptom status
- Guidelines recommend consideration for surgery in asymptomatic patients with abnormal response to exercise (symptoms, <20 mm Hg increase in BP, ST depression, and/or complex ventricular arrhythmias).[21]

DOBUTAMINE STRESS ECHOCARDIOGRAPHY (DSE)

* Employed in patients with AS, depressed LVEF with two primary goals
* DSE can help distinguish severe stenosis from pseudo (flow dependent) AS.[22]
* DSE can help to identify patients with pre-operative cardiac reserve (increase in stroke volume by >20%, or in mean transvalvular gradient of 10 mm Hg) as this subset of patients with low EF tends to have better outcomes (surgical mortality of 6% vs. 33%).[23]

CARDIAC CATHETERIZATION AND ANGIOGRAPHY

* Catheterization is used to assess coronary anatomy (prior to surgery).
* Catheterization used to confirm/clarify diagnosis, severity by determining transvalvular gradient (simultaneous aortic, LV pressures are most accurate) and calculation of AVA by Gorlin formula or Hakki formula.
* The gradient is dependent on transvalvular flow, so errors occur in patients with low cardiac output.
* Dobutamine can be used to distinguish pseudostenosis from true anatomically severe AS.

Management: General Principles

* Identify patients that warrant surgery with close monitoring for onset of symptoms.
* Medical therapy has a limited role in providing a survival benefit or slowing progression.
* Symptomatic severe AS should be referred for surgery: Mortality high without surgery[16]; age-corrected survival after surgery is near normal.[24]
* Patients with asymptomatic severe AS generally have a good prognosis,[25] but there is a risk of sudden death (~ 2%) and of irreversible myocardial damage.[25,26]
* Identify subset of asymptomatic severe AS patients at risk for SCD and/or onset symptoms that would require surgery in the near future.
* Patients at highest risk for symptom onset/needing surgery in the short term include: Peak aortic velocity >4 m/s;[24] Severe calcification of the aortic valve;[10] Rapid progression of aortic velocity (increase of >0.3 m/s per year).[10]
* Exercise testing: A negative test has a strong negative predictive value (85%-87%) for event-free survival[20] but is positively predictive (79%) only in physically active patients <70 years old.[21]
* No randomized controlled data support the strategy of referring "high-risk" patients with asymptomatic severe AS for AVR, but this is a Class II recommendation (see Table 12-3).

Medical Therapy

* Antibiotic prophylaxis is indicated if high risk for endocarditis (see Chapter 13).[26]
* Afterload agents are considered to be contraindicated because of concern over hemodynamic collapse (supporting data is lacking).

TABLE 12-3   Indications for AVR in AS

Class I

1. Symptomatic patients with severe AS
2. Patients with severe AS undergoing CABG, or surgery on aorta/other valves
3. Patients with severe AS and depressed LVEF (<50%)

Class II

1. Patients with moderate AS undergoing CABG, surgery of the aorta, or other heart valves (IIa)
2. Asymptomatic patients with severe AS and
   – Abnormal response to exercise (symptoms or hypotension) (IIb)
   – Critical AS (valve area <0.6 cm², mean gradient >60 mm Hg, aortic jet velocity >5 m/s)
   – High likelihood of rapid progression (age, calcification, CAD)

Adapted from AHA/ACC 2006 Guidelines on Management of Patients with Valvular Heart Disease.[1]

- Considered to be contraindicated because of concern over hemodynamic collapse (supporting data is lacking)
- Afterload reducing agents have been shown to be beneficial in patients with severe AS and bw EF[27] and decompensated CHF.[28]
- ACE inhibitors are well tolerated.[29]
- Studies on effect of ACE inhibitors on progression of AS have yielded conflicting results.[31,32]
- Data on the role of statins in slowing progression of AS is conflicting.
- Recent retrospective data suggest statins may slow progression of AS.[33–35]
- A single randomized controlled trial showed no effect of statins on progression of AS.[36]
- Several randomized controlled trials of statins in AS are pending.

Surgical Management: Aortic Valve Replacement (AVR)

- AVR is the only effective treatment for symptomatic AS.
- Symptoms/high risk features are the chief indications for AVR.
- Operative mortality for AVR ~5% to 30% depending on the patient population
- Age itself is not an absolute contraindication to AVR.[37,38]
- Predictors of higher operative mortality and lower late survival: CHF, low LVEF, chronic kidney disease, urgent procedures, and need for concomitant CABG or MVR[39]
- Outcomes similar in patients with preserved LV function and with moderate LV dysfunction
- Patients with low EF/low gradient AS have higher operative mortality (20%).[40,41]
- Provocative testing (DSE) can identify patients with contractile reserve; this subgroup may have better surgical outcomes.[23]

- Surgical mortality is very high (30%–50%) in patients with severe AS and decompensated heart failure who are taken directly to surgery[42] (balloon valvuloplasty and medical optimization are important bridge therapies).
- In patients with severe AS who need surgical intervention, but are poor candidates, percutaneous AVR may represent a safe, viable alternative.[43]

AORTIC REGURGITATION

Background
- Aortic regurgitation (AR) is due to ineffective coaptation of aortic cusps.
- The prevalence of chronic AR increases with age; the majority of patients with AR have trace or mild AR.[44]
- Grading of severity is based on several qualitative and/or quantitative measures. (See Table 12-4.)

Etiology
- AR can be due to primary valvular disease and/or aortic pathology (see Table 12-5).
- AR can be acute or chronic, and the clinical presentation of each entity is distinct.
- Chronic AR is more common than acute AR.
- Acute AR is commonly caused by endocarditis, aortic dissection, and trauma.
- Chronic AR is usually due to degenerative, aortic root, congenital abnormalities.

Pathophysiology

ACUTE AR
- Large regurgitant volume into a nondilated LV leads to an abrupt increase in LV end diastolic pressure (LVEDP).

TABLE 12-4 Grading of severity of AR

Severity of AR	Mild	Moderate	Severe
Qualitative			
Angiographic grade	1+	2+	3+
Doppler central jet width	<25% LVOT	25%–65% LVOT	>65%
Vena contracta width (cm)	<0.3	0.3–0.6	LVOT >0.6
Quantitative			
Regurgitant volume (mL/beat)	<30	30–59	>60
Regurgitant fraction	<30%	30–49	>50
Regurgitant orifice area (cm^2)	<0.1	0.1–0.29	>0.3

Adapted from AHA/ACC 2006 Guidelines on Management of Patients with Valvular Heart Disease.[1]

TABLE 12-5 Etiology of AR

Etiology	Notes
Primary valve disease	
1. **Degenerative AR**	Associated with ascending aortic aneurysm
2. **Congenital abnormalities**	Bicuspid valve (increased risk of aortic coarctation, root dilatation, and dissection)
	VSD
	Subvalvular AS
	Rare abnormalities: Congenital valve fenestration, unicommissural/quadricusp valve
3. **Rheumatic heart disease**	Thick, retracted leaflets with central regurgitation
4. **Endocarditis**	Leaflet perforation/tears, perivalvular abscess with abnormal aorta-LV communication
5. **Rare causes**	Complications of valvuloplasty, balloon dilation
– Trauma	Appetite suppressants (fenfluramine)
– Drugs	Including antiphospholipid syndrome
– Connective tissue disease	
– Chest radiation	
Primary aortic disease	
1. **Annulus/Aortic root dilatation**	
– Idiopathic root dilatation	Isolated aortic root pathology
– Annulo-aortic ectasia	Dilation present in ∼80%, AR present in ∼30%[45]
– Marfan syndrome	Dilation present in ∼30%[45]
– Ehlers-Danlos syndrome	
– Osteogenesis imperfecta	
2. **Aortitis**	
– Infectious	Syphilitic aortitis now a rare etiology
– Inflammatory diseases	Ankylosing spondylitis, RA, SLE, Behcet disease, giant cell and Takayasu arteritis, relapsing polychondritis, Reiters syndrome
3. **Aortic dissection**	

- Compensatory tachycardia usually insufficient to maintain cardiac output
- Poor hemodynamic tolerance: LVEDP equalizes with diastolic aortic pressure with subsequent pulmonary edema and cardiogenic shock.

CHRONIC AR
- Combined volume and pressure overload on the LV
- Volume overload due to regurgitant volume
- Pressure overload due to increased afterload (hypertension [HTN] from increased aortic stroke volume)
- Three compensatory mechanisms initially preserve cardiac output: Increased LV end diastolic volume; increased chamber compliance; LVH (eccentric/concentric).

- Compensated phase can last for years/decades.
- Eventually, progressive LV dilation and LV systolic dysfunction lead to CHF.

History
- Patients with acute AR present with marked dyspnea and pulmonary edema.
- Patients with chronic AR can be asymptomatic for many years.
- Angina without structural coronary artery disease is due to decreased coronary perfusion (due to high LVEDP).
- Exertional dyspnea is the most common presenting symptom in chronic AR (late stage).
- Syncope and sudden cardiac death are rare in absence of other symptoms.

Natural History
- Progression of AR results from complex interplay of multiple variables.
- Mild AR: Minimal data on natural history; Most patients with mild AR probably do not progress to severe AR.
- Moderate to severe AR
  - A. Asymptomatic patients with normal systolic function
    - Rate of progression (decrease in EF, symptoms, death) of 4% to 6% per year[46,47]
    - Up to one fourth develop systolic dysfunction or die suddenly.[46–49]
    - Predictors of progression: Age, LV dimensions at end systole (LVIDs) and LV dimension at end diastole (LVIDd), and LVEF during exercise[46,47,48,49–51]
    - Unlike AS, onset of symptoms is not the only important factor
  - B. Asymptomatic patients with systolic dysfunction
    - Rate of progression to symptoms of $\sim$ 25%/year[52–54]
    - Majority will need AVR in 2 to 3 years
  - C. Symptomatic patients
    - No contemporary studies, but outcomes are poor with medical therapy
    - High mortality rates: Angina – mortality of $\sim$ 10%/year; heart failure – mortality of $\sim$ 25%/year[55–57]

Physical Exam
- The high-frequency decrescendo blowing diastolic murmur is heard best over the left lower sternal border (LLSB) through stethoscope's diaphragm with patient sitting upright during forced expiration.
- Murmurs that are louder over right lower scapular border (RLSB) are more likely due to aortic root/ascending aorta pathology, rather than primary valve abnormalities.

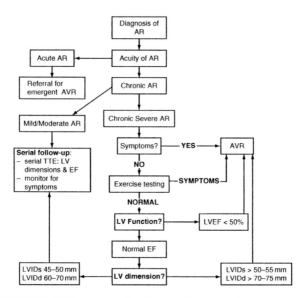

FIGURE 12-2 Management algorithm: aortic regurgitation

- Duration of murmur correlates with severity (mild AR – short murmur; severe AR – typically holodiastolic).
- In acute AR, the diastolic murmur and peripheral signs (see Table 12-6) may be absent (the only clue may be absent S2 with hypotension/pulmonary edema).
- Austin Flint murmur (mid-late diastolic rumble that resembles MS – due to vibration from AR jet striking the mitral valve)
- Pulse: High-amplitude, rapidly collapsing pulse (waterhammer pulse)

Lab Exams and Imaging
- Chest x-ray can be normal or demonstrate pulmonary edema, cardiomegaly, or dilated aorta.
- ECG shows LAD, LVH and signs of LV diastolic volume overload (high QRS amplitude and tall T waves with ST depression), and conduction abnormalities.

Echocardiography
- Assessment of anatomy of aortic leaflets, aortic root, LV size/function, and severity of AR

TABLE 12-6	Auscultatory and peripheral findings in severe AR: A glossary of eponyms

Sign	Description
Austin Flint murmur[a]	Low-pitched apical mid-diastolic rumble
Corrigan pulse[a]	High-amplitude, abruptly collapsing pulse
Duroziez sign[a]	To-and-fro bruit over femoral artery
Hill sign[a]	>40 mm HgΔ between popliteal and brachial pressures
Mayne sign	>15 mm Hg drop in SBP with arm elevation pressure
Traube sign	Loud systolic "pistol shots" over the femoral artery
Quincke pulse	Exaggerated reddening and blanching of nail beds
Mueller sign	Visible pulsations of the uvula
de Musset sign	Visible bobbing of the head

[a]Signs identified in a recent review of physical findings in AR as the most significant findings based on a review of available literature (peer-reviewed journals and classic text books). Babu A, et al. *Ann Intern Med.* 2003;138:736–742.[58]

- Estimation of severity is based on color flow and Doppler parameters (Table 12-4)
- Supportive findings:
  - Early mitral valve closure by M-Mode (can be masked by tachycardia)
  - AR pressure half time: Mild >500 milliseconds and severe <200 milliseconds (confounded by filling volumes and diastolic function)
  - Holodiastolic flow reversal in descending aorta reflective of at least moderately severe AR
- Recommendations for serial studies in asymptomatic patients
  - Mild AR and normal LV size and function: Every 2 to 3 years
  - Patients with LV dilation: Every 6 to 12 months
  - Patients with advanced LV dilation (LVIDs >50 mm, LVIDd >70 mm): Risk of progression 10%–20%/year;[46] studies every 4–6 mos.
  - Associated aortic root disease: Monitoring of aortic root size

Cardiac Catheterization and Angiography
- Useful in initial assessment if echocardiography is suboptimal[1]
- Aortography provides semiquantitative estimates of severity of AR
- Coronary angiogram pre-operatively to diagnose co-existing CAD
- Routinely performed in men >35 years and premenopausal women >45 years with risk factors

Management: General Principles
- Close monitoring for onset of symptoms and evidence of changes in LV size and function

* Appropriate for referral for surgery
* Unlike AS, monitoring for onset of symptoms alone is NOT sufficient.
* LV size and systolic function have a significant impact on prognosis.
* Surgery is indicated in symptomatic patients, and in patients with severe LV chamber dilation and/or LV dysfunction (even in the absence of symptoms).
* Medical therapy has limited role.
* The optimal surgical option depends on the etiology of AR and aortic pathology.

Medical Therapy

* Antibiotic prophylaxis is indicated in high risk patients with AR (prosthetic valves, prior endocarditis, unrepaired congenital heart disease—please see Chapter 13[26]).
* **Acute AR**
  – The role of medical therapy is limited if there is evidence of heart failure.
  – Negative chromotropes should be avoided; they lengthen diastole and may increase regurgitant fraction and precipitate hemodynamic collapse.
  – Nitroprusside and inotropic agents can serve as temporizing measures.
  – Intra-aortic balloon pulsation (IABP) is contra-indicated.
* **Chronic severe asymptomatic AR with preserved LV function and size**
  – The goal of medical therapy is to reduce systolic blood pressure and mitigate the afterload mismatch.
  – Vasodilator therapy with hydralazine[59] and nifedipine[60] have been shown in small randomized control trials to decrease LVIDd and increase LVEF.
  – Nifedipine delayed surgery when compared with digoxin,[61] but recent trials showed no effect of nifedipine or enalapril on timing of surgery.[62]

Surgical Management: Aortic Valve Replacement (AVR)

* Acute AR requires emergent surgical intervention.
* In chronic AR, AVR is the only effective treatment for symptomatic patients.
* Indications for AVR in asymptomatic patients:

  – Depressed LVEF ($<50\%$)[63]
  – If LVEF is normal, excessive ventricular dilation (marker of incipient systolic dysfunction): LVIDs >55 mm[64] or LVIDd >70 mm[65]
  – In patients with established LV dysfunction, the majority of patients improve although some may have irreversible dysfunction: In short-term follow-up (14–18 months), 72% of patients with severe asymptomatic AR and LV dysfunction who underwent AVR had stable or improved LVEF.[66]

TABLE 12-7	Indications for AVR in AR

Class I

1. Symptomatic patients with severe AR
2. Patients with severe AR undergoing CABG, or surgery on aorta/other valves
3. Asymptomatic patients with severe AR and LV dysfunction (LVEF <50%)

Class II

1. Asymptomatic patients with severe AR with normal LVEF but severe LV dilation (LVIDd 70–75 mm and LVIDs 50–55 mm)
2. Patients with moderate AR undergoing CABG or surgery of the aorta or other heart valves

Adapted from AHA/ACC 2006 Guidelines on Management of Patients with Valvular Heart Disease.[1]

MITRAL REGURGITATION

Background
- Dysfunction of any part of the valve apparatus (leaflets, annulus, chordae tendineae, papillary muscles, LV) can lead to mitral regurgitation (MR).
- Prevalence of MR increases with age (1.3-fold increase per decade).[44]
- Acute MR leads to rapid decline; chronic MR is tolerated for prolonged period (see Table 12-8).

Etiology
- MR can be due either to primary disease of the valve apparatus or to cardiac/systemic/genetic diseases that affect the valve apparatus.
- The most common etiologies in patients with chronic severe MR include mitral valve prolapse (MVP), ischemic MR, rheumatic heart disease, and endocarditis.[67–72] (see Table 12-9)
- Acute MR can result from structural (papillary muscle dysfunction/rupture, chordal rupture due to myxomatous changes) and infectious (endocarditis, acute rheumatic fever) etiologies.

Pathophysiology
ACUTE MR
- The regurgitant volume in LV produces an abrupt increase in LVEDP and left atrial pressure.
- Higher preload (abrupt volume overload), lower afterload (systolic runoff into LA)[73] and compensatory increased LV contractility.
- There is a modest increase in cardiac output, but overall LV function declines: Majority of the stroke volume is directed to the LA.
- Pulmonary edema, cardiogenic shock can develop due to poor forward flow.

CHRONIC MR
- MR causes pure volume overload, unlike AR (combined volume/pressure load).

TABLE 12-8	Grading of severity of MR		
Severity of MR	Mild	Moderate	Severe
Qualitative			
Angiographic grade	1+	2+	3+-4+
Doppler central jet width	<20% LA area	20%–40% LA area	>40% LA area
Vena contracta width (cm)	<0.3	0.3–0.69	>0.7
LA/LV size			Enlarged
Quantitative			
Regurgitant volume (mL/beat)	<30	30–59	>60
Regurgitant fraction	<30%	30–49	>50
Regurgitant orifice area (cm^2)	<0.2	0.2–0.39	>0.4

Adapted from AHA/ACC 2006 Guidelines on Management of Patients with Valvular Heart Disease.[1]

TABLE 12-9	Etiology of MR
Etiology	Notes
Primary mitral apparatus disease	
1. MVP (myxomatous disease)	
2. Rheumatic heart disease	Acute rheumatic fever and chronic rheumatic valvular disease
3. Endocarditis	MR due to perforation, incomplete coaptation, chordal rupture
4. Congenital lesions	Cleft anterior leaflet (associated with ASD and other congenital heart disease)
	Leaflet fenestration
	Parachute mitral valve (associated with endocardial cushion defects and transposition)
5. Mitral annular calcification	Degenerative changes of leaflets
	Increased annular rigidity
6. Idiopathic chordal rupture	Associated MR is typically mild to moderate
7. Trauma	Surgical/percutaneous valvuloplasty
8. Drugs	Methysergide
9. Radiation therapy	
Secondary MR	
1. Cardiac disease	
– CAD	Papillary muscle rupture
	Transmural myocardial infarction (MI)
	Ischemic regional dysfunction
	Global ventricular dysfunction

– Dilated cardiomyopathy	Incomplete closure due to annular dilation from LV chamber dilation
– Hyphertrophic cardiomyopathy (HCM)	Systolic anterior motion (SAM) leads to MR with elongated leaflets
– Endomyocardial fibrosis	
2. Systemic disease	
– Systemic lupus erythematosus (SLE)	
– Hypereosinophilic syndrome	
– Amyloidosis	25% have significant MR
– Rheumatoid arthritis	
– Marfan syndrome	
– Ehlers Danlos (Type I and III)	
– Scleroderma	
– Pseudoxanthoma elasticum	
– Ankylosing spondylitis	Anterior leaflet long/redundant with MR

* Compensatory mechanisms (LVH and increased contractility/compliance) initially preserve cardiac output.
* The compensated phase can persist for years, with high-normal LVEF.
* LA dilation, RV dilation/dysfunction due to pulmonary hypertension
* Over time, progressive LV dysfunction, LV dilation leads to CHF.[74,75]

History
* Clinical history depends on the etiology and acuity of onset of MR.
* Symptoms include the insidious onset of dyspnea on exertion and exercise intolerance and progress to overt CHF.
* MR may manifest symptoms in the context of hemodynamic stress such as pregnancy, infection, and new onset AF with rapid ventricular response.
* Acute MR (due to chordal rupture or endocarditis) presents with acute decompensated CHF.

Natural History
* The clinical course depends on the etiology of MR, the status of both ventricles and of the left atrium.
* The compensated phase of MR may last for several years (up to 10-15 years).[76]
* There are limited data on the progression of mild/moderate MR, with wide individual variability.[77]
* In MVP/MR, the 5-year event-free rates are 85% to 95% for mild-moderate MR.[78]
* There is a high likelihood (5%–10%) of developing symptoms/LV dysfunction in severe asymptomatic MR.[79–82]

- Patients with asymptomatic severe MR have a mortality rate of ~ 5%/year.[76,79]
- LVEF is the best validated predictor of outcome.
- When LVEF <60%, survival after MVR is lower.[83]
- When symptoms develop, survival is improved with surgical intervention.[76,84]

Physical Exam
- Auscultation
- Soft S1 with normal S2 early on; later a loud P2 appears when pulmonary HTN develops.
- S3 may be present independent of presence of LV failure.
- The holosystolic murmur is loudest over apex.
- Posterolateral jets (radiating to axilla/back) are heard with ischemic disease, anterior leaflet abnormalities, and dilated cardiomyopathy.
- Anterior jets (radiating to sternum/base/carotids mimicking AS) are heard with posterior leaflet prolapse.
- Maneuvers to distinguish from AS: Handgrip (increased afterload) augments MR and softens AS (lower transvalvular gradients); AS murmer increases post PVC while MR murmer changes; AS but not MR heard over right clavicle.
- In chronic MR, the intensity of the murmur correlates with severity.
- In acute MR, 50% of patients have no murmur.[85]
- Midsystolic and late systolic murmur if mitral valve prolapse is present

Lab Exams and Imaging
- Chest x-ray can be normal early, shows left atrial enlargement and cardiomegaly later in the course of disease.
- ECG findings are nonspecific (LAE, LVH, AF).
- Echocardiography is useful for assessing:
  - Severity (See Table 12-8.)
  - Anatomic mechanism of MR
  - Assessment of anatomy of mitral valve apparatus (especially 3-D echo)
  - Evaluation of LV size and systolic function
  - Evaluation of left atrial size and pulmonary artery pressures
  - Assessment of options for valve repair versus replacement
- TEE is useful if TTE images are suboptimal, and pre-operatively for mapping to determine type of repair and likelihood of successful repair.
- Estimation of severity is based on a combination of color flow and Doppler (see table).
- Systolic flow reversal in pulmonary veins indicates moderate-to-severe MR.
- Recommendations for serial studies (in the absence of symptoms): mild MR and normal LV size and function, Every 2 to 3 years; severe MR, Every 6 to 12 months

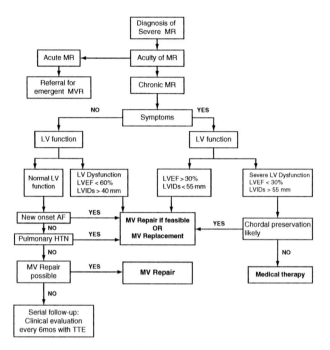

FIGURE 12-3 Management algorithm: mitral regurgitation

Exercise Testing
* Provides objective data on symptoms and change in exercise tolerance
* Measurement of PA pressures and severity of MR during exercise is useful.
* The precise role of exercise testing in determining need for surgery is not clearly defined because many of the patients studied were already symptomatic.

Cardiac Catheterization and Angiography
* Useful if there is a discrepancy between clinical and noninvasive data[1]
* Performed pre-operatively to screen for CAD if cardiac risk factors are present
* Ventriculography provides semiquantitative estimates of MR severity.
* Right heart catheterization is performed to assess right-sided filling pressures, PA pressures, and PCWP.

Management: General Principles
* Close monitoring for onset of symptoms and evidence of changes in LV size and function
* Appropriate referral for surgery (see Table 12-10)
* LV size and systolic function have a significant impact on prognosis (see Table 12-11).
* Surgery is indicated in symptomatic patients, and patients with LV chamber dilation and/or LV dysfunction (even in the absence of symptoms).
* Medical therapy has limited role.
* Optimal surgical option depends on the etiology of MR.

Medical Therapy
* Antibiotic prophylaxis if indicated (see endocarditis chapter)[26]
* **Acute MR**
    - The role of medical therapy is limited to stabilization prior to surgery.
    - Main goals: (a) ↓ MR; (b) ↑ forward cardiac output; (c) ↓ pulmonary congestion
    - Normotensive patients: Nitroprusside[86]
    - Hypotensive patients: Nitroprusside and inotropic agent (dobutamine)
    - IABP to decrease afterload and increase forward CO
* **Chronic severe asymptomatic MR with preserved LV function and size**
    - There has been sustained interest in vasodilator therapy, but there are no data to support its clinical efficacy in delaying surgery.[87]
    - Vasodilator therapy is most effective in MR secondary to LV dilation.[88] Nitroprusside and hydralazine have been shown to decrease MR, LV, and increase forward cardiac output.
    - ACE inhibitors do not consistently reduce severity of primary MR.[88-90]

Surgical Intervention
* Acute MR requires emergent surgical intervention.
* In chronic MR, surgery is the only effective treatment for symptomatic patients.
* Three types of MV operations are possible for correction of MR:
    - MV repair
    - MV replacement with preservation of chordal preservation
    - MV replacement (MVR)
* Indications for surgical intervention in chronic severe MR:
    1. Symptomatic patients (NHYA Class II-IV): LVEF 30–60%; no severe LV dysfunction (LVEF < 30% or LVIDs < 55 mm)
    2. Asymptomatic patients: LVIDs > 40 mm and/or LVIDd > 75 mm; new onset AF; pulmonary HTN(>50 mm Hg at rest or >60 mm with exercise)

TABLE 12-10   Indications for surgical intervention in MR

Class I

1. Acute symptomatic severe MR
2. Chronic severe MR
   - Symptomatic patients (NYHA Class II-IV) in *absence* of severe LV dysfunction (LVEF <30% and/or LVIDs >55 mm)
   - Asymptomatic patients with mild-moderate LV dysfunction (LVEF 30%-60%, LVIDs >40 mm)
3. MV repair preferable to MVR if repair is feasible

Class II

1. Asymptomatic chronic severe MR
   - New onset AF
   - Pulmonary HTN (>50 mm Hg at rest, >60 mm Hg with exercise)
   - MV repair in patients with preserved LV function (LVEF >60% and LVIDs <40 mm) if likelihood of successful repair >90%
   - MV repair in patients with severe LV dysfunction (LVEF <30% and/or LVIDs >40 mm) if likelihood of successful repair >90%

Adapted from AHA/ACC 2006 Guidelines on Management of Patients with Valvular Heart Disease.[1]

- MV repair preserves the native valve apparatus, although technically more difficult, leads to better post-operative LV function and survival.[91–97]
- Reoperation rates are similar to MVR (10% at 10 years).[98]
- MVR is associated with higher operative mortality and less favorable outcomes compared to surgery for AS, AR, or MS, as well as MV repair.
- Overall surgical mortality with MVR is 5-10%(higher for ischemic than for rheumatic/ myxomatous MR) and overall survival rates poor (5-85% at 5 years).[99]

TABLE 12-11   Severity of MS

Severity of MR	Mild	Moderate	Severe
Parameter			
Mean gradient (mm Hg)	<5	5–10	>10
PA systolic pressure (mm Hg)	<30	30–50	>50
Valve area (cm^2)	>1.5	1.0–1.5	<1.0

Adapted from AHA/ACC 2006 Guidelines on Management of Patients with Valvular Heart Disease.[1]

- MVR with preservation of chordal apparatus is better post-operative LV function and survival.[99–101,102]
- MVR with resection of chordal apparatus is rarely performed given the better outcomes with preserved chordal apparatus (necessary in rheumatic cases where the valve apparatus is deformed).

MITRAL STENOSIS

Background
- The normal MV area is 4 to 6 cm^2.
- A diastolic transmitral gradient and symptoms appear at valve areas < 2 cm^2.[103]
- Rheumatic carditis is the predominant cause of MS.
- MS found in ∼ 40% of patients with chronic rheumatic heart disease.[104,105]
- The ratio of women to men in isolated MS is 2:1.[104,105]
- Grading severity is based on valve area, gradient, and degree of pulmonary HTN.

Etiology
- Rheumatic heart disease is the major cause of acquired MS; congenital MS is rare (see Table 12-12).
- Other rare causes of acquired mitral inflow obstruction include atrial myxoma, valve thrombus, mucopolysaccharidosis, and severe mitral annular calcification.

Pathophysiology
- Obstruction leads to increased diastolic pressure between the left atrium and LV.
- Transmitral gradients increase with more severe obstruction and higher flow rates across the MV (fever, anemia, exercise, and co-existing MR).
- Progressive limitation of cardiac output with rise in left atrial pressure (LAP) and pulmonary HTN.
- Increased LAP leads to chamber enlargement and low-velocity flow.
- AF develops due to high LAP and rheumatic insults to the left atrium.
- AF further reduces flow velocity (especially in LA appendage), leading to a very high risk of thrombus.
- Pulmonary HTN develops due to high LAP and pulmonary vascular remodeling.
- Chronic pulmonary HTN can lead to RVH, RV dilation, and RV failure.
- LV systolic function is typically preserved, but forward stroke volume may be impaired due to impaired diastolic filling from the MS or RV overload.

History
- Insidious onset of fatigue and exercise intolerance due to decreased forward cardiac output

TABLE 12-12 Etiology of MS

Etiology	Notes
Acquired causes	
1. Rheumatic heart disease	Rheumatic heart disease is the most common
2. Carcinoid heart disease	cause of acquired MS. Fusion of one/both com-
3. Fabry disease	missures, with thickening/fibrosis calcification
4. Mucopolysaccharidosis	of valves. Other valves involved in rheumatic
5. Rheumatoid arthritis	heart disease in one third of cases (tricuspid
6. SLE	disease and AR most frequently)
7. Atrial tumor	
8. Large vegetation	
9. Whipple disease	
10. Gout	
Congenital	
1. Supravalvular ring	Congenital abnormalities frequently associated
2. Mitral valve abnormalities	with other left ventricular outflow tract (LVOT) obstruction and ventricular septal defect (VSD)

- Dyspnea on exertion, paroxysmal nocturnal dyspnea (PND), and pulmonary edema from accompanying elevated LAP
- Right heart failure (edema, ascites) can arise from pulmonary HTN.
- AF and/or embolic events can be the first manifestations of MS.
- Less common presentations include hemoptysis (severe MS) and hoarseness (compression of the recurrent laryngeal nerve from a giant LA)
- Recurrent pulmonary infections are common in severe MS.
- Hemodynamic stresses (anemia, infection, pregnancy) are common precipitants.

Natural History

- Stable course initially, followed by accelerated progression in later life[104–106]
- Rate of progression 0.09 to 0.32 cm^2/year (slower in United States and Europe[107,108])
- The interval between acute rheumatic fever and symptomatic MS is ~15 years.[109]
- Once symptoms develop, another ~10 years before symptoms become disabling[104]
- Overall, the 10-year survival of untreated patients is 50% to 60%,[105,106] but 0% to 15% once disabling symptoms develop.[104–106,110,111]
- Mortality in MS is due to progressive systemic/pulmonic congestion, thromboembolism, and infection (higher rates of pneumonia).

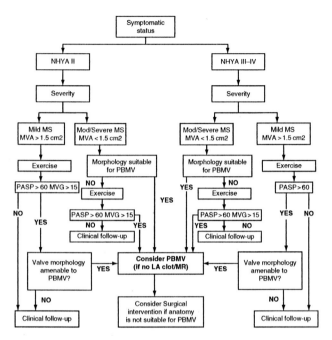

FIGURE 12-4 Management algorithm: aortic stenosis. PBMV, percu-laneous balloon mitral valvuloplasty; PASP, pulmonary artery systolic pressure; MVG, mitral valve gradient.

Physical Exam

* JVP: Normal or elevated with prominent CV wave from TR
* Loud snapping S1
* Opening snap (medium-high pitch) not heard with heavy calcification, mixed mitral disease, pulmonary HTN, RV dilation
* A shorter S2-OS interval indicative of more severe disease
* The diastolic rumbling murmur is best heard in the midprecordial area.
* In severe MS, the murmur is pandiastolic.
* TR and pulmonic regurgitation murmur (Graham-Steele murmur) if pulmonary HTN is present

Lab Exams and Imaging

* Chest x-ray is normal early in disease but LAE and pulmonary HTN develop later.
* ECG commonly shows LAE and AF (RVH, RAD if pulmonary HTN).

- Echocardiography
  - Quantification of stenosis severity (see Table 12-11) based on *valve area*, *transmitral gradient*, and *pulmonary HTN*
  - Valve morphology (restricted leaflet opening and doming of anterior leaflet/immobility of posterior leaflet) and evaluation for MR, as well as other valve disease (associated rheumatic AS in 17%, AR in 8%, and TR in 38%)[112]
  - Rule out other causes of obstruction (LA myxoma, parachute MV, Cor triatrium).
- Wilkins valve score (leaflet thickening, calcification, mobility, subvalvular involvement) to determine suitability for balloon valvulotomy
- Formal exercise testing with measurement of transmitral gradient and PA pressures may help determine timing of intervention.
- Serial follow-up of asymptomatic patients: Severe MS – yearly TTE; moderate MS – TTE every 1 to 2 years; mild MS – every 3 to 5 years
- TEE if TTE is inadequate or to rule out thrombus prior to percutaneous intervention.

Cardiac Catheterization and Angiography
- Useful if there is discrepancy between clinical and noninvasive data
- Gorlin formula can be used to determine MVA and PVR.
- Angiography pre-operatively to screen for CAD if cardiac risk factors present

Management: General Principles
- Identification of patients who will benefit from intervention (see Table 12-13)
- Periodic evaluation: Subjective assessment of symptom status and objective assessment of LV function/size and exercise tolerance
- Annual follow-up with the indication for chest x-ray, ECG, or TTE based on severity of MS
- Holter monitoring in patients with palpitations in the absence of documented AF

Medical Therapy
- Medical therapy cannot address mechanical obstruction to mitral inflow.
- Asymptomatic patients with mild MS in sinus rhythm need no specific therapy.
- Patients with AF or atrial flutter (30%–40%) have high risk for thromboembolism and need anticoagulation, but data specific to MS is limited.[113–115]
- Patients with MS/AF should have efforts to restore sinus rhythm (balloon valvulotomy or cardioversion with adjunctive antiarrhythmic therapy).
- Anticoagulation may be considered for asymptomatic patients with severe MS NSR, if LA dimension >55 mm Hg even in sinus rhythm.[1]

TABLE 12-13 Indications for intervention in MS

Indications for percutaneous mitral balloon valvulotomy

Class I

1. Moderate/severe MS with NYHA II-IV symptoms with favorable morphology if no atrial thrombus or moderate/severe MR
2. Asymptomatic moderate/severe MS with pulmonary HTN (>50 mm Hg at rest, >60 mm Hg with exercise) if morphology is favorable and no concomitant left atrial thrombus/significant MR

Class II

1. Symptomatic (NYHA II-IV) moderate/severe MS with nonpliable calcified valve if NOT a candidate for surgical intervention or high risk for surgery
2. Symptomatic patients (NYHA II-IV) with valve area >1.5 cm^2 if there is evidence of pulmonary HTN (>50 mm Hg at rest and >60 mm Hg with exercise)
3. Asymptomatic patients with moderate/severe MS with favorable morphology with new onset AF (if no left atrial thrombus/significant MR)

Class III

1. Mild MS
2. Mild MS with left atrial thrombus, significant MR

Indications for surgery

Class I

1. Symptomatic moderate/severe MS with acceptable operative risk when (a) percutaneous mitral valvulotomy is not available or contraindicated or (b) unfavorable anatomy is present
2. Symptomatic patients with moderate/severe MS with concomitant severe MR

Class II

1. MV replacement for symptomatic patients with severe MS and severe pulmonary HTN who are not candidates for percutaneous intervention or surgical commisurotomy
2. MV repair for asymptomatic patients with moderate or severe MS who have had recurrent embolic events while receiving adequate anticoagulation with favorable anatomy for repair

Class III

1. MV repair is not indicated in mild MS

Adapted from AHA/ACC 2006 Guidelines on Management of Patients with Valvular Heart Disease.[1]

- Endocarditis and rheumatic fever prophylaxis
- Avoidance of strenuous activity (increases in HR lead to high LAP) but low-level aerobic activity is recommended to prevent deconditioning
- Beta blockers are useful for patients with exertional symptoms (blocks tachycardia).
- Salt restriction and diuretics for patients with pulmonary congestion

Percutaneous Intervention: Mitral Balloon Valvulotomy

* The preferred procedure in select patients with pliable, noncalcified valves and minimal fusion of the subvalvular apparatus
* In these patients, immediate and long-term results (3–7 years) are comparable to surgical commissurotomy.[116–118]
* The mean valve area usually doubles, with a 50% decrease in transmitral gradient in the immediate postprocedure period.
* Long term follow-up (3–7 years): 90% of patients free of events remain in NYHA I-II.
* Outcomes are heavily dependent on operator experience.
* Complications include severe MR (2%–10%), large residual ASD (5%), LV perforation (0.5%–4%), embolic events (0.5%–3%), and MI (0.5%).[103]
* Postprocedure: Baseline TTE at 72 hours and consideration for immediate surgery if either severe MR or large residual ASD is present
* Relative contraindications to PMV include: Significant (3-4+) MR; Left atrial thrombus; Unfavorable valve anatomy (calcied valve, high Wilkins score)

Surgical Intervention

* Surgical commissurotomy or MVR are options.
* Surgical commissurotomy can be done open or closed.
* Closed procedures are procedures of choice in developing countries whereas open procedures are preferred in developed countries.
* Open procedures allow direct inspection of the valve.
* Commissurotomy is usually combined with left atrial appendage resection.
* Long-term outcomes are clearly better for commissurotomy than for medical therapy.[118–121]
* Five-year event-free survival rates of 80% to 90% with re-operation rate of 4% to 7%
* MVR is an acceptable option in patients who are not candidates for surgical commissurotomy or percutaneous valvulotomy.
* The risk of surgery is lower in young patients with normal LV function, good functional status, and no comorbid diseases such as CAD.
* Peri-operative mortality ranges from less than 5% to 20%.
* Preservation of the mitral valve apparatus is preferable (to preserve LVEF) but often not possible in rheumatic MS.
* Complications include valve thrombosis, valve dehiscence, valve malfunction, and embolic events.

RIGHT-SIDED VALVE DISEASE

Background

* Due to primary valve disease or pulmonary HTN

- Primary valve abnormalities are usually congenital and diagnosed early.
- In adults, right-sided valve disease is usually due to pulmonary HTN.
- Less common acquired causes include trauma, endocarditis, and drugs.
- Difficult to assess impact on the RV (complex RV dimensions make quantification of the RV function difficult)

TRICUSPID VALVE DISEASE

Tricuspid Regurgitation
- Primary TR is due to primary valve abnormalities.
- Secondary TR is due to conditions that affect the RV (pulmonary HTN, chronic obstructive pulmonary disease (COPD), RV dysplasia, ischemia, posttransplant state).
- Primary causes include congenital etiologies (Ebstein anomaly) and acquired conditions (rheumatic heart disease, myxomatous degeneration, endocarditis, carcinoid, endomyocardial fibrosis, trauma, and iatrogenic causes).
- Secondary causes are more common.
- Moderate-to-severe TR is frequently well tolerated.
- There is little information on natural history.
- Patients s/p TV resection tolerate severe TR well for several years.[122]
- Other concomitant valve disease is usually present and usually dictates clinical course.
- Isolated severe TR presents with fatigue, exercise intolerance, and RV failure.
- Physical exam: Prominent jugular V wave, jugular venous distension, hepatomegaly +/− pulsatility, a classic holosystolic murmur at the LLSB that increases with inspiration (murmur heard only 20% of cases)[123,124]
- Echocardiography: Severe TR with systolic flow reversal in hepatic veins
- Patients with mild-to-moderate TR do not require any specific therapy.
- Medical therapy is designed to control peripheral venous congestion with diuretics.
- Surgical intervention considered for patients with *severe TR*
- The most common procedure is annuloplasty (surgical plication vs. complete ring vs. semicircular ring).
- Many patients have residual TR, and 40% develop TS.[125]
- TV replacement is performed only if annuloplasty is not feasible or fails.
- Variable outcomes
- Heart block is the main complication.
- High risk of valve thrombosis with mechanical valves (4%–30%)[126]

Tricuspid Stenosis
- Primarily due to rheumatic heart disease[127]; only 3% to 5% of patients with rheumatic heart disease have tricuspid stenosis (TS)

- Rare etiologies: Carcinoid, congenital defects, endocarditis, and Whipple disease
- Majority of patients have concomitant mitral disease and TR
- There are limited data on natural history, but TS usually takes a slowly progressive course.
- Clinical presentation with fatigue, dyspnea, edema
- Physical exam notable: OS, diastolic murmur at RLSB (murmur often inaudible)
- ECG shows AF in 90% of cases
- Chest x-ray: RAE
- Echocardiography
- Rheumatic involvement with commissural fusion and diastolic doming
- Findings can be subtle.
- Doppler evaluation
- Medical therapy with diuretics often ineffective
- Optimal surgical intervention for severe TS: Direct tricuspid commissurotomy +/− annuloplasty

Pulmonic Stenosis

- The majority of cases (95%) are due to congenital abnormalities; 85% occur as an isolated defect, but can occur in association with other congenital defects (tetralogy of Fallot, pulmonary artery aneurysms).
- Other rare etiologies include carcinoid disease and rheumatic heart disease.
- Patients with mild PS (gradient <50 mm Hg) are rarely symptomatic, and outcomes are good without surgical intervention.[128−129]
- Severe PS (>80 mm Hg) typically leads to fatigue and dyspnea on exertion, and right heart failure and surgery may be beneficial.[129]
- Clinical outcomes for patients with moderate stenosis (50-80 mm Hg)
- Overall survival at 25 years was 96% in a natural history study,[129] and predictors of poor outcome include presence of symptoms, cardiomegaly on chest x-ray, hypotension, and elevated right sided pressures.
- Physical examination
- Crescendo-decrescendo systolic murmur loudest at left upper sternal border (LUSB)
- Radiation to the suprasternal notch and left neck
- Loud late-peaking murmur is suggestive of severe obstruction.
- An ejection click may be heard.
- Echocardiography
- Thickened pulmonic leaflets with doming in systole
- Severity based on transpulmonic velocity and gradient (severe: Velocity >1.2 m/s and gradient >80 mm Hg)
- Pulmonary HTN
- Cardiac catheterization is not typically required unless clinical data and noninvasive data are discordant.

- There is a limited role for medical therapy.
- The intervention of choice for severe PS is balloon valvuloplasty, which has low morbidity and mortality and generally leads to decrease in gradient by two thirds.
- Accompanying subvalvular stenosis often regresses after valvuloplasty.

Pulmonary Regurgitation
- Small degrees of PR present in normal adults.
- Pathologic PR occurs after intervention for congenital heart disease (tetralogy of Fallot), and can also be due to rheumatic heart disease, carcinoid disease, or endocarditis.
- PA/annular dilatation due to pulmonary HTN, Marfan syndrome, or volume overload (as seen in renal failure) can also lead to PR.
- Patients with mild PR have a benign course.
- Patients with moderate/severe PR can develop chronic RV volume overload, dilation, and failure.
- Physical exam
- The soft, diastolic, decrescendo diastolic murmur over LUSB may be difficult to hear.
- May be accompanied by PS murmur
- Echocardiogram
- Abnormal diastolic flow in right ventricular outflow tract (RVOT)
- Holodiastolic flow reversal in PA
- Severity graded qualitatively (0–4+) on extent of color flow
- RV dilation and dysfunction
- No specific therapy is required for mild PR.
- Surgical intervention should be considered for severe PR with evidence of progressive RV dilation/dysfunction.
- Surgical procedure of choice is placement of a homograft conduit, although a prosthetic valve can be used as well.
- RV size and functional status can improve after surgery.[130]

REFERENCES

1. Bonow RO, et al., ACC/AHA 2006 guidelines for the management of patients with valvular heart disease. *Circulation*, 2006. 114(5): p. e84–231.
2. Otto, CM, Valvular aortic stenosis: disease severity and timing of intervention. *J Am Coll Cardiol*, 2006. 47(11): p. 2141–2151.
3. Griffith, MJ, et al., Inaccuracies in using aortic valve gradients alone to grade severity of aortic stenosis. *Br Heart J*, 1989. 62(5): p. 372–378.
4. Passik, CS, et al., Temporal changes in the causes of aortic stenosis: a surgical pathologic study of 646 cases. *Mayo Clin Proc*, 1987. 62(2): p. 119–123.

5. Carlson, RG, et al., Radiation-associated valvular disease. *Chest*, 1991. 99(3): p. 538–545.

6. Marcus, ML, et al., Decreased coronary reserve: a mechanism for angina pectoris in patients with aortic stenosis and normal coronary arteries. *N Engl J Med*, 1982. 307(22): p. 1362–1366.

7. Schwartz, LS, et al., Syncope and sudden death in aortic stenosis. *Am J Cardiol*, 1969. 23(5): p. 647–658.

8. Richards, AM, et al., Syncope in aortic valvular stenosis. *Lancet*, 1984. 2(8412): p. 1113–1116.

9. Pellikka, PA, et al., The natural history of adults with asymptomatic, hemodynamically significant aortic stenosis. *J Am Coll Cardiol*, 1990. 15(5): p. 1012–1017.

10. Rosenhek, R, et al., Predictors of outcome in severe, asymptomatic aortic stenosis. *N Engl J Med*, 2000. 343(9): p. 611–617.

11. Horstkotte, D and F Loogen, The natural history of aortic valve stenosis. *Eur Heart J*, 1988. 9 Suppl E: p. 57–64.

12. Bogart, DB, et al., Progression of aortic stenosis. *Chest*, 1979. 76(4): p. 391–396.

13. Nitta, M, et al., Noninvasive evaluation of the severity of aortic stenosis in adults. *Chest*, 1987. 91(5): p. 682–687.

14. Ng, AS, et al., Hemodynamic progression of adult valvular aortic stenosis. *Cathet Cardiovasc Diagn*, 1986. 12(3): p. 145–150.

15. Nestico, PF, et al., Progression of isolated aortic stenosis: analysis of 29 patients having more than 1 cardiac catheterization. *Am J Cardiol*, 1983. 52(8): p. 1054–1058.

16. Ross, J, Jr and E Braunwald, Aortic stenosis. *Circulation*, 1968. 38(1 Suppl): p. 61–67.

17. Lim, P, et al., Predictors of outcome in patients with severe aortic stenosis and normal left ventricular function: role of B-type natriuretic peptide. *Eur Heart J*, 2004. 25(22): p. 2048–2053.

18. Bergler-Klein, J, et al., Natriuretic peptides predict symptom-free survival and postoperative outcome in severe aortic stenosis. *Circulation*, 2004. 109(19): p. 2302–2308.

19. Currie, PJ, et al., Continuous-wave Doppler echocardiographic assessment of severity of calcific aortic stenosis: a simultaneous Doppler-catheter correlative study in 100 adult patients. *Circulation*, 1985. 71(6): p. 1162–1169.

20. Baumgartner, H, et al., "Overestimation" of catheter gradients by Doppler ultrasound in patients with aortic stenosis: a predictable manifestation of pressure recovery. *J Am Coll Cardiol*, 1999. 33(6): p. 1655–1661.

21. Das, P, H Rimington, and J Chambers, Exercise testing to stratify risk in aortic stenosis. *Eur Heart J*, 2005. 26(13): p. 1309–1313.

22. Wu, WC, LA Ireland, and A Sadaniantz, Evaluation of aortic valve disorders using stress echocardiography. *Echocardiography*, 2004. 21(5): p. 459–466.
23. Quere, JP, et al., Influence of preoperative left ventricular contractile reserve on postoperative ejection fraction in low-gradient aortic stenosis. *Circulation*, 2006. 113(14): p. 1738–1744.
24. Otto, CM, et al., Prospective study of asymptomatic valvular aortic stenosis. Clinical, echocardiographic, and exercise predictors of outcome. *Circulation*, 1997. 95(9): p. 2262–2270.
25. Lund, O, Preoperative risk evaluation and stratification of long-term survival after valve replacement for aortic stenosis. Reasons for earlier operative intervention. *Circulation*, 1990. 82(1): p. 124–139.
26. Wilson, W, et al., Prevention of infective endocarditis. *Circulation*, 2007. 116(15): p. 1736–1754.
27. Ikram, H, et al., Hemodynamic effects of nitroprusside on valvular aortic stenosis. *Am J Cardiol*, 1992. 69(4): p. 361–366.
28. Khot, UN, et al., Nitroprusside in critically ill patients with left ventricular dysfunction and aortic stenosis. *N Engl J Med*, 2003. 348(18): p. 1756–1763.
29. Chockalingam, A, et al., Safety and efficacy of angiotensin-converting enzyme inhibitors in symptomatic severe aortic stenosis. *Am Heart J*, 2004. 147(4): p. E19.
30. Rosenhek, R, et al., Statins but not angiotensin-converting enzyme inhibitors delay progression of aortic stenosis. *Circulation*, 2004. 110(10): p. 1291–1295.
31. O'Brien, KD, et al., Angiotensin-converting enzyme inhibitors and change in aortic valve calcium. *Arch Intern Med*, 2005. 165(8): p. 858–862.
32. Newby, DE, SJ Cowell, and NA Boon, Emerging medical treatments for aortic stenosis: statins, angiotensin converting enzyme inhibitors, or both? *Heart*, 2006. 92(6): p. 729–734.
33. Novaro, GM, et al., Effect of hydroxymethylglutaryl coenzyme a reductase inhibitors on the progression of calcific aortic stenosis. *Circulation*, 2001. 104(18): p. 2205–2209.
34. Bellamy, MF, et al., Association of cholesterol levels, hydroxymethylglutaryl coenzyme-A reductase inhibitor treatment, and progression of aortic stenosis in the community. *J Am Coll Cardiol*, 2002. 40(10): p. 1723–1730.
35. Aronow, WS, et al., Association of coronary risk factors and use of statins with progression of mild valvular aortic stenosis in older persons. *Am J Cardiol*, 2001. 88(6): p. 693–695.
36. Cowell, SJ, et al., A randomized trial of intensive lipid-lowering therapy in calcific aortic stenosis. *N Engl J Med*, 2005. 352(23): p. 2389–2397.

37. Chiappini, B, et al., Outcome after aortic valve replacement in octogenarians. *Ann Thorac Surg*, 2004. 78(1): p. 85–89.
38. Salazar, E, et al., Aortic valve replacement in patients 70 years and older. *Clin Cardiol*, 2004. 27(10): p. 565–570.
39. Edwards, FH, et al., Prediction of operative mortality after valve replacement surgery. *J Am Coll Cardiol*, 2001. 37(3): p. 885–892.
40. Sharony, R, et al., Aortic valve replacement in patients with impaired ventricular function. *Ann Thorac Surg*, 2003. 75(6): p. 1808–1814.
41. Monin, JL, et al., Low-gradient aortic stenosis: operative risk stratification and predictors for long-term outcome: a multicenter study using dobutamine stress hemodynamics. *Circulation*, 2003. 108(3): p. 319–324.
42. Hutter, AM, Jr, et al., Aortic valve surgery as an emergency procedure. *Circulation*, 1970. 41(4): p. 623–627.
43. Webb, JG, et al., Percutaneous transarterial aortic valve replacement in selected high-risk patients with aortic stenosis. *Circulation*, 2007. 116(7): p. 755–763.
44. Singh, JP, et al., Prevalence and clinical determinants of mitral, tricuspid, and aortic regurgitation. *Am J Cardiol*, 1999. 83(6): p. 897–902.
45. Hwa, J, et al., The natural history of aortic dilatation in Marfan syndrome. *Med J Aust*, 1993. 158(8): p. 558–562.
46. Bonow, RO, et al., Serial long-term assessment of the natural history of asymptomatic patients with chronic aortic regurgitation and normal left ventricular systolic function. *Circulation*, 1991. 84(4): p. 1625–1635.
47. Borer, JS, et al., Prediction of indications for valve replacement among asymptomatic or minimally symptomatic patients with chronic aortic regurgitation and normal left ventricular performance. *Circulation*, 1998. 97(6): p. 525–534.
48. Scognamiglio, R, G Fasoli, and S Dalla Volta, Progression of myocardial dysfunction in asymptomatic patients with severe aortic insufficiency. *Clin Cardiol*, 1986. 9(4): p. 151–156.
49. Siemienczuk, D, et al., Chronic aortic insufficiency: factors associated with progression to aortic valve replacement. *Ann Intern Med*, 1989. 110(8): p. 587–592.
50. Tarasoutchi, F, et al., Ten-year clinical laboratory follow-up after application of a symptom-based therapeutic strategy to patients with severe chronic aortic regurgitation of predominant rheumatic etiology. *J Am Coll Cardiol*, 2003. 41(8): p. 1316–1324.
51. Dujardin, KS, et al., Mortality and morbidity of aortic regurgitation in clinical practice. A long-term follow-up study. *Circulation*, 1999. 99(14): p. 1851–1857.
52. Ishii, K, et al., Natural history and left ventricular response in chronic aortic regurgitation. *Am J Cardiol*, 1996. 78(3): p. 357–361.

53. Goldschlager, N, et al., The natural history of aortic regurgitation. A clinical and hemodynamic study. *Am J Med*, 1973. 54(5): p. 577–588.

54. Reimold, SC, et al., Progressive enlargement of the regurgitant orifice in patients with chronic aortic regurgitation. *J Am Soc Echocardiogr*, 1998. 11(3): p. 259–265.

55. Hegglin, R, H Scheu, and M Rothlin, Aortic insufficiency. *Circulation*, 1968. 38(1 Suppl): p. 77–92.

56. Spagnuolo, M, et al., Natural history of rheumatic aortic regurgitation. Criteria predictive of death, congestive heart failure, and angina in young patients. *Circulation*, 1971. 44(3): p. 368–380.

57. Rapaport, E, Natural history of aortic and mitral valve disease. *Am J Cardiol*, 1975. 35(2): p. 221–227.

58. Babu, AN, SM Kymes, and SM Carpenter Fryer, Eponyms and the diagnosis of aortic regurgitation: what says the evidence? *Ann Intern Med*, 2003. 138(9): p. 736–742.

59. Greenberg, B, et al., Long-term vasodilator therapy of chronic aortic insufficiency. A randomized double-blinded, placebo-controlled clinical trial. *Circulation*, 1988. 78(1): p. 92–103.

60. Scognamiglio, R, et al., Long-term nifedipine unloading therapy in asymptomatic patients with chronic severe aortic regurgitation. *J Am Coll Cardiol*, 1990. 16(2): p. 424–429.

61. Scognamiglio, R, et al., Nifedipine in asymptomatic patients with severe aortic regurgitation and normal left ventricular function. *N Engl J Med*, 1994. 331(11): p. 689–694.

62. Evangelista, A, et al., Long-term vasodilator therapy in patients with severe aortic regurgitation. *N Engl J Med*, 2005. 353(13): p. 1342–1349.

63. Forman, R, BG Firth, and MS Barnard, Prognostic significance of preoperative left ventricular ejection fraction and valve lesion in patients with aortic valve replacement. *Am J Cardiol*, 1980. 45(6): p. 1120–1125.

64. Bonow, RO, Asymptomatic aortic regurgitation: indications for operation. *J Card Surg*, 1994. 9(2 Suppl): p. 170–173.

65. Turina, J, et al., Improved late survival in patients with chronic aortic regurgitation by earlier operation. *Circulation*, 1984. 70(3 Pt 2): p. I147–I152.

66. Bonow, RO, et al., Reversal of left ventricular dysfunction after aortic valve replacement for chronic aortic regurgitation: influence of duration of preoperative left ventricular dysfunction. *Circulation*, 1984. 70(4): p. 570–579.

67. Agozzino, L, et al., Surgical pathology of the mitral valve: gross and histological study of 1288 surgically excised valves. *Int J Cardiol*, 1992. 37(1): p. 79–89.

68. Hanson, TP, BS Edwards, and JE Edwards, Pathology of surgically excised mitral valves. One hundred consecutive cases. *Arch Pathol Lab Med*, 1985. 109(9): p. 823–828.
69. Amlie, JP, F Langmark, and O Storstein, Pure mitral regurgitation. Etiology, pathology and clinical patterns. *Acta Med Scand*, 1976. 200(3): p. 201–208.
70. Falco, A, et al., Etiology and incidence of pure mitral insufficiency: a morphological study of 926 native valves. *Cardiologia*, 1990. 35(4): p. 327–330.
71. Olson, LJ, et al., Surgical pathology of the mitral valve: a study of 712 cases spanning 21 years. *Mayo Clin Proc*, 1987. 62(1): p. 22–34.
72. Turri, M, et al., Surgical pathology of disease of the mitral valve, with special reference to lesions promoting valvar incompetence. *Int J Cardiol*, 1989. 22(2): p. 213–219.
73. Ross, J, Jr, Afterload mismatch and preload reserve: a conceptual framework for the analysis of ventricular function. *Prog Cardiovasc Dis*, 1976. 18(4): p. 255–264.
74. Urabe, Y, et al., Cellular and ventricular contractile dysfunction in experimental canine mitral regurgitation. *Circ Res*, 1992. 70(1): p. 131–147.
75. Mulieri, LA, et al., Myocardial force-frequency defect in mitral regurgitation heart failure is reversed by forskolin. *Circulation*, 1993. 88(6): p. 2700–2704.
76. Delahaye, JP, et al., Natural history of severe mitral regurgitation. *Eur Heart J*, 1991. 12 Suppl B: p. 5–9.
77. Enriquez-Sarano, M, et al., Progression of mitral regurgitation: a prospective Doppler echocardiographic study. *J Am Coll Cardiol*, 1999. 34(4): p. 1137–1144.
78. Zuppiroli, A, et al., Natural history of mitral valve prolapse. *Am J Cardiol*, 1995. 75(15): p. 1028–1032.
79. Ling, LH, et al., Clinical outcome of mitral regurgitation due to flail leaflet. *N Engl J Med*, 1996. 335(19): p. 1417–1423.
80. Rosen, SE, et al., Natural history of the asymptomatic/minimally symptomatic patient with severe mitral regurgitation secondary to mitral valve prolapse and normal right and left ventricular performance. *Am J Cardiol*, 1994. 74(4): p. 374–380.
81. Enriquez-Sarano, M, et al., Quantitative determinants of the outcome of asymptomatic mitral regurgitation. *N Engl J Med*, 2005. 352(9): p. 875–883.
82. Rosenhek, R, et al., Outcome of watchful waiting in asymptomatic severe mitral regurgitation. *Circulation*, 2006. 113(18): p. 2238–2244.
83. Enriquez-Sarano, M, et al., Echocardiographic prediction of left ventricular function after correction of mitral regurgitation: results and clinical implications. *J Am Coll Cardiol*, 1994. 24(6): p. 1536–1543.

84. Munoz, S, et al., Influence of surgery on the natural history of rheumatic mitral and aortic valve disease. *Am J Cardiol*, 1975. 35(2): p. 234–242.

85. Sutton, GC and E Craige, Clinical signs of severe acute mitral regurgitation. *Am J Cardiol*, 1967. 20(1): p. 141–144.

86. Greenberg, BH and SH Rahimtoola, Usefulness of vasodilator therapy in acute and chronic valvular regurgitation. *Curr Probl Cardiol*, 1984. 9(4): p. 1–46.

87. Tischler, MD, M Rowan, and MM LeWinter, Effect of enalapril therapy on left ventricular mass and volumes in asymptomatic chronic, severe mitral regurgitation secondary to mitral valve prolapse. *Am J Cardiol*, 1998. 82(2): p. 242–245.

88. Levine, HJ and WH Gaasch, Vasoactive drugs in chronic regurgitant lesions of the mitral and aortic valves. *J Am Coll Cardiol*, 1996. 28(5): p. 1083–1091.

89. Host, U, et al., Effect of ramipril on mitral regurgitation secondary to mitral valve prolapse. *Am J Cardiol*, 1997. 80(5): p. 655–658.

90. Marcotte, F, et al., Effect of angiotensin-converting enzyme inhibitor therapy in mitral regurgitation with normal left ventricular function. *Can J Cardiol*, 1997. 13(5): p. 479–485.

91. Enriquez-Sarano, M, et al., Congestive heart failure after surgical correction of mitral regurgitation. A long-term study. *Circulation*, 1995. 92(9): p. 2496–2503.

92. Duran, CG, et al., Conservative operation for mitral insufficiency: critical analysis supported by postoperative hemodynamic studies of 72 patients. *J Thorac Cardiovasc Surg*, 1980. 79(3): p. 326–337.

93. Yacoub, M, et al., Surgical treatment of mitral regurgitation caused by floppy valves: repair versus replacement. *Circulation*, 1981. 64(2 Pt 2): p. II210–II216.

94. David, TE, DE Uden, and HD Strauss, The importance of the mitral apparatus in left ventricular function after correction of mitral regurgitation. *Circulation*, 1983. 68(3 Pt 2): p. II76–II82.

95. Perier, P, et al., Comparative evaluation of mitral valve repair and replacement with Starr, Bjork, and porcine valve prostheses. *Circulation*, 1984. 70(3 Pt 2): p. I187–I192.

96. Goldman, ME, et al., Mitral valvuloplasty is superior to valve replacement for preservation of left ventricular function: an intraoperative two-dimensional echocardiographic study. *J Am Coll Cardiol*, 1987. 10(3): p. 568–575.

97. Tischler, MD, et al., Mitral valve replacement versus mitral valve repair. A Doppler and quantitative stress echocardiographic study. *Circulation*, 1994. 89(1): p. 132–137.

98. Mohty, D, et al., Very long-term survival and durability of mitral valve repair for mitral valve prolapse. *Circulation*, 2001. 104(12 Suppl 1): p. I1–I7.

99. Okita, Y, et al., Comparative evaluation of left ventricular performance after mitral valve repair or valve replacement with or without chordal preservation. *J Heart Valve Dis*, 1993. 2(2): p. 159–166.

100. Hennein, HA, et al., Comparative assessment of chordal preservation versus chordal resection during mitral valve replacement. *J Thorac Cardiovasc Surg*, 1990. 99(5): p. 828–836; discussion 836–837.

101. Rozich, JD, et al., Mitral valve replacement with and without chordal preservation in patients with chronic mitral regurgitation. *Circulation*, 1992. 86(6): p. 1718–1726.

102. Horskotte, D, et al., The effect of chordal preservation on late outcome after mitral valve replacement. *J Heart Valve Dis*, 1993. 2(2): p. 150–158.

103. Gorlin, R and SG Gorlin, Hydraulic formula for calculation of the area of the stenotic mitral valve, other cardiac valves, and central circulatory shunts. I. *Am Heart J*, 1951. 41(1): p. 1–29.

104. Wood, P, An appreciation of mitral stenosis. I. Clinical features. *Br Med J*, 1954. 1(4870): p. 1051–1063; contd.

105. Rowe, JC, et al., The course of mitral stenosis without surgery: ten- and twenty-year perspectives. *Ann Intern Med*, 1960. 52: p. 741–749.

106. Olesen, KH, The natural history of 271 patients with mitral stenosis under medical treatment. *Br Heart J*, 1962. 24: p. 349–357.

107. Dubin, AA, et al., Longitudinal hemodynamic and clinical study of mitral stenosis. *Circulation*, 1971. 44(3): p. 381–389.

108. Gordon, SP, et al., Two-dimensional and Doppler echocardiographic determinants of the natural history of mitral valve narrowing in patients with rheumatic mitral stenosis: implications for follow-up. *J Am Coll Cardiol*, 1992. 19(5): p. 968–973.

109. Horstkotte, D, R Niehues, and BE Strauer, Pathomorphological aspects, aetiology and natural history of acquired mitral valve stenosis. *Eur Heart J*, 1991. 12 Suppl B: p. 55–60.

110. Selzer, A and KE Cohn, Natural history of mitral stenosis: a review. *Circulation*, 1972. 45(4): p. 878–890.

111. van den Brink, RB, et al., The value of Doppler echocardiography in the management of patients with valvular heart disease: analysis of one year of clinical practice. *J Am Soc Echocardiogr*, 1991. 4(2): p. 109–120.

112. Sagie, A, et al., Echocardiographic assessment of mitral stenosis and its associated valvular lesions in 205 patients and lack of association with mitral valve prolapse. *J Am Soc Echocardiogr*, 1997. 10(2): p. 141–148.

113. Abernathy, WS and PW Willis, 3rd, Thromboembolic complications of rheumatic heart disease. *Cardiovasc Clin*, 1973. 5(2): p. 131–175.

114. Adams, GF, et al., Cerebral embolism and mitral stenosis: survival with and without anticoagulants. *J Neurol Neurosurg Psychiatry*, 1974. 37(4): p. 378–383.

115. Hwang, JJ, et al., Significance of left atrial spontaneous echo contrast in rheumatic mitral valve disease as a predictor of systemic arterial embolization. *Am Heart J*, 1994. 127(4 Pt 1): p. 880–885.

116. Pan, M, et al., Factors determining late success after mitral balloon valvulotomy. *Am J Cardiol*, 1993. 71(13): p. 1181–1185.

117. Cohen, DJ, et al., Predictors of long-term outcome after percutaneous balloon mitral valvuloplasty. *N Engl J Med*, 1992. 327(19): p. 1329–1335.

118. Dean, LS, et al., Four-year follow-up of patients undergoing percutaneous balloon mitral commissurotomy. *J Am Coll Cardiol*, 1996. 28(6): p. 1452–1457.

119. Dahl, JC, P Winchell, and CW Borden, Mitral stenosis. A long term postoperative follow-up. *Arch Intern Med*, 1967. 119(1): p. 92–97.

120. Ellis, LB, et al., Fifteen-to twenty-year study of one thousand patients undergoing closed mitral valvuloplasty. *Circulation*, 1973. 48(2): p. 357–364.

121. John, S, et al., Closed mitral valvotomy: early results and long-term follow-up of 3724 consecutive patients. *Circulation*, 1983. 68(5): p. 891–896.

122. Frater, RW, Surgical management of endocarditis in drug addicts and long-term results. *J Card Surg*, 1990. 5(1): p. 63–67.

123. Muller, O and J Shillingford, Tricuspid incompetence. *Br Heart J*, 1954. 16(2): p. 195–207.

124. Sepulveda, G and DS Lukas, The diagnosis of tricuspid insufficiency; clinical features in 60 cases with associated mitral valve disease. *Circulation*, 1955. 11(4): p. 552–563.

125. Duran, CM, Tricuspid valve surgery revisited. *J Card Surg*, 1994. 9(2 Suppl): p. 242–247.

126. Jugdutt, BI, et al., Long-term survival after tricuspid valve replacement. Results with seven different prostheses. *J Thorac Cardiovasc Surg*, 1977. 74(1): p. 20–27.

127. Kitchin, A and R Turner, Diagnosis and Treatment of Tricuspid Stenosis. *Br Heart J*, 1964. 26: p. 354–379.

128. Johnson, LW, et al., Pulmonic stenosis in the adult. Long-term follow-up results. *N Engl J Med*, 1972. 287(23): p. 1159–1163.

129. Nugent, EW, et al., Clinical course in pulmonary stenosis. *Circulation*, 1977. 56(1 Suppl): p. I38–I47.

130. Therrien, J, et al., Pulmonary valve replacement in adults late after repair of tetralogy of fallot: are we operating too late? *J Am Coll Cardiol*, 2000. 36(5): p. 1670–1675.

CHAPTER 13

Endocarditis

TODD L. KIEFER, FRED A. LOPEZ, AND RANDALL VAGELOS

NATIVE VALVE ENDOCARDITIS

Etiologies[1,2]

- *Staphylococcus aureus*: Increasing prevalence; *Streptococcus viridans*; *Streptococcus* species: *S. mitis, S. mutans, S. bovis, S. sanguis*; Coagulase-negative *Staphylococcus* species: *Staphylococcus lugdunensis* is quite virulent; *Enterococcus* species; Gram-negative bacilli; Fungi: *Candida* and *Aspergillus* species
- Other less common organisms, which are often "culture negative": HACEK organisms (*Haemophilus* species, *Actinobacillus actinomycetemcomitans*, *Cardiobacterium hominis*, *Eikenella corrodens*, *Kingella kingae*), *Abiotrophia* species, *Bartonella quintana*, *Bartonella henselae*, *Tropheryma whipplei*, *Legionella*, *Coxiella burnetii*, *Brucella* species, *Chlamydia psittaci*, *Mycoplasma*, *Neisseria gonorrhoeae*

Clinical Presentation[3]

Fever, weight loss, fatigue, anorexia, arthritis/arthralgias, myalgias, skin manifestations, cough, mental status changes, headache

Risk Factors

Mitral valve prolapse (most common), other valvular abnormalities, hemodialysis, indwelling vascular catheters, intravenous drug use

Differential Diagnosis/Endocarditis Mimics[4]

Atrial myxoma, carcinoid valve disease, myxomatous valve degeneration, papillary fibroelastoma, Lambl excrescence, ruptured chordae, thrombus or stitch after valvular surgery, eosinophilic heart disease, acute rheumatic fever, pulmonary embolus, CVA.

PHYSICAL EXAM

Cardiac auscultation for evidence of new heart murmur (in particular, murmur of valvular regurgitation), Janeway's lesions, Osler's nodes (painful), splinter hemorrhages, Roth spots, skin petechiae, oral petechiae, conjunctival hemorrhage, splenomegaly, clubbing, S3 gallop, lung crackles.

Electrocardiogram (ECG)

Evaluate for prolonged P-R interval or high-grade A-V block suggestive of aortic perivalvular abscess, or evidence of other new conduction abnormalities

DIAGNOSIS[5]

Modified Duke Criteria for definite infective endocarditis: 2 major criteria or; 1 major and 3 minor criteria or; 5 minor criteria

Major criteria: blood culture positive for typical organism from two separate blood cultures or persistent culture positive from specimens greater than 12 hours apart or all of 3 or a majority of greater than 4 separate cultures with an organism consistent with endocarditis, new valvular regurgitation, echocardiogram positive for endocarditis (oscillating mass, abscess, or partial dehiscence of prosthetic valve), evidence of endocardial involvement, blood culture positive for Coxiella burnetti or IgG titer > 1:800.

Minor criteria: temperature > 38° C, vascular (Janeway's lesions, emboli, mycotic aneurysm), immunologic (Osler's nodes, Roth's spots, glomerulonephritis, positive rheumatoid factor), positive blood culture not meeting major criteria or serological data supporting infection with organism known to cause endocarditis, predisposing heart condition or intravenous drug use.

Laboratory evaluation:[6] Blood cultures prior to antibiotics; if initial cultures are negative (approximately 10%) and diagnosis is still suspected, alert lab to hold for fastidious organisms (HACEK organisms); May also be associated with leukocytosis, anemia, and/or microscopic hematuria

Chest radiograph: May reveal septic pulmonary emboli from right-sided endocarditis

Echocardiography[7-9]: Transsthoracic echo: Starting point for suspected native valve endocarditis: Sensitivity: 32% to 63%; Specificity: 98% to 100%; Transesophageal echo: Next step if transthoracic echocardiogram (TTE) nondiagnostic and endocarditis is still suspected; First step in evaluation of patient with prosthetic valve (see section below), high clinical suspicion, or anticipated difficulty imaging with TTE; Also perform pre-operatively if patient will undergo valve surgery: Sensitivity: 94% to 100%; Specificity: 98% to 100%; Additional considerations for transesophageal echocardiography (TEE): Enhanced ability to detect myocardial abscess, aneurysm, fistula

TREATMENT [10]

Early cardiothoracic surgery consultation and evaluation with coordination of care involving infectious diseases and cardiology consultants.

Antibiotic regimens: See reference 10 for dosing regimens.

* Penicillin-sensitive *Streptococcus viridans* and *S. bovis*: Penicillin G or ceftriaxone for 4 weeks OR Vancomycin for 4 weeks with penicillin allergy
* Penicillin-resistant *Streptococcus viridans* and *S. bovis*: Penicillin G or ceftriaxone for 4 weeks with the addition of gentamicin for 2 weeks OR Vancomycin for 4 weeks with penicillin allergy
* Penicillin-sensitive *Enterococcus*: Ampicillin for 4–6 weeks with the addition of gentamicin for 4–6 weeks; penicillin G for 4–6 weeks with the addition of gentamicin for 4–6 weeks; vancomycin and gentamicin for 6 weeks with penicillin allergy
* Oxacillin-sensitive *Staphylococcus*: Nafcillin or oxacillin for 6 weeks +/− 3–5 days of gentamicin; cefazolin for 6 weeks with penicillin allergy (not ananphylaxis)
* Oxacillin-resistant *Staphylococcus*: Vancomycin for 6 weeks
* HACEK endocarditis: Ceftriaxone or ampicillin/sulbactam or ciprofloxacin (ampicillin/ceftriaxone allergy) for 6 weeks
* Inpatient parenteral antibiotics first 2 weeks of treatment when risk of embolism and other complications is highest, then selection of lower-risk patients for outpatient parenteral therapy based on published guidelines[8]
* High risk for outpatient therapy: congestive heart failure (CHF), arrhythmia, altered mental status, perivalvular abscess, aortic valve disease, prosthetic valve disease, infection with *S. aureus, Streptococcus pneumoniae, Haemophilus influenzae, Neisseria meningitides* or *N. gonorrhoeae*, betahemolytic Strep, gram-negative organisms, or fungal organism[11]

Indications for surgery:[10] **Class I:** heart failure secondary to valve stenosis or insufficiency, aortic or mitral insufficiency with elevated left ventricular end-diastolic or left atrial pressures, aortic insufficiency with mitral valve pre-closure, fungal endocarditis, infection with highly resistant organism, heart block, abscess, fistula formation, or mitral leaflet perforation. **Class IIa:** recurrent embolic events, persistent vegetation with appropriate antimicrobial therapy. **Class IIb:** mobile vegetation > 10 mm.

OUTCOMES

Overall mortality of 10% to 20% for hospitalized patients, 30% to 40% 1-year mortality[12]

* Right-sided endocarditis: Mortality less than 10%[13]
* Significant increase in 6-month survival with valve replacement surgery for left-sided endocarditis using current criteria for valve replacement (16% vs. 33%); most significant decrease in mortality seen in patients with evidence of moderate to severe CHF (14% vs. 51%)[14]

Five Predictors of 6-Month Mortality with Left-sided Endocarditis[12]

* Comorbid medical conditions, Altered mental status, Moderate to severe CHF, Organism other than *S. viridans*, Medical therapy without valve replacement

Predictors of Early In-hospital Mortality[15] (based on data collected during initial 7 days of hospitalization)

* Diabetes mellitus, *S. aureus* endocarditis, Embolic event, Elevated APACHE II score

Complications[4,16,17]

* Embolism: 20% to 40% of cases of endocarditis, of these cerebral - 62%, splenic - 49%, renal - 22%, *coronary* - 2%
* Risk of embolization increases with the size and mobility of the vegetation and mitral valve presents a greater risk than aortic valve vegetation
* Abscess (local cardiac or metastatic)
* Vertebral osteomyelitis
* Septic arthritis
* Immune-complex glomerulonephritis
* Renal infarction
* Mycotic aneurysm
* Fistula: Most commonly between paravalvular infection and sinuses of Valsalva, aorta, or pulmonary artery: Associated with > 50% mortality
* Valvular perforation
* Congestive heart failure
* Cardiogenic shock
* Arrhythmias (A-V block): Increased mortality associated with infranodal conduction block
* Sepsis

Relapse Rate[1]

Most common in 4 weeks following termination of antibiotics: Higher relapse rates with *Enterococcus*, *S. aureus*, Gram-negative bacilli, fungal pathogens

INFECTIVE ENDOCARDITIS ASSOCIATED WITH INTRAVENOUS DRUG USE[13]

* **Etiologies**: *Staphylococcus* species, *Pseudomonas* species, Fungi (*Candida* species)
* **Clinical presentation**: Fever, cough, pleuritic chest pain, hemoptysis
* Most commonly involves right-sided valves, can be left-sided or both left- and right-sided

- **Chest radiograph**: May demonstrate multiple pulmonary infiltrates suggestive of septic pulmonary emboli
- **Treatment**:[13] Two-week duration of nafcillin and gentamicin for uncomplicated right-sided infection (i.e., absence of aortic/mitral valve involvement, not MRSA, no high-level gentamicin resistance, no extrapulmonary evidence of metastatic infection, no renal insufficiency
- **Predictors of worse outcome**:[13] HIV infection
- Increasing mortality with low CD4 levels (<200 cells/mL^3)

PACEMAKER OR IMPLANTED CARDIOVERTER DEFIBRILLATOR (ICD)-ASSOCIATED ENDOCARDITIS[18–21]

- **Etiology**: *S. aureus* (most common less than 1 month postplacement), coagulase-negative Staphylococci, Streptococci, *Candida*, *Peptostreptococcus* species, *Propionibacterium acnes*, Enterobacteriaceae, *Pseudomonas*
- Cleveland Clinic series of device endocarditis in 123 patients with pacemaker or ICD: 68% coagulase-negative *Staphylococcus*, 24% *S. aureus*, 17% Gram-negative rods, 13% polymicrobial[18]
- **Clinical Presentation**: May have erythema or pain over device pocket, fever, chills, malaise, anorexia
- **Treatment**: Complete system explant and antibiotic therapy
- In one series, 41% mortality with antibiotic therapy alone compared with 19% mortality with antibiotics and pacemaker removal
- **Duration**: At least 4 to 6 weeks of parenteral antibiotics based on sensitivity of specific organism isolated
- **Timing of reimplantation of device**: Literature varies with recommendations of 1 to 6 weeks delay with patient remaining afebrile and with negative repeat blood cultures. Plan for reimplantation on contralateral side.
- If pacemaker dependent, place temporary pacing wire with change every 5–10 days until permanent device can be placed as outlined above
- If at high risk for lethal arrhythmia, patient may wear external defibrillator vest until ICD can be replaced.

PROSTHETIC VALVE ENDOCARDITIS[22]

- 4% risk infectious endocarditis with mechanical prosthetic valve >5 years
- Higher incidence of early prosthetic valve endocarditis with surgery performed during active infective endocarditis
- Aortic PVE more common than mitral PVE
- Early: Within 2 months of surgery up to 1 year (nosocomial)
- **Etiologies**: *S. aureus*, coagulase-negative Staphylococci, Gram-negative bacilli, fungi, Enterococci, diphtheroids: Late—After 2 to 12 months postoperation (community-acquired)

- **Etiologies:** *Streptococcus* species, coagulase-negative Staphylococci, *S. aureus*, Enterococci (i.e., similar to non-IVDU associated native valve endocarditis microbiology)
- **Predisposing factors:** Wound infection, intravascular catheter-associated infection, urinary tract infection, pneumonia
  - **Treatment:**[10] Early cardiothoracic surgery consultation and evaluation with coordination of care involving infectious diseases and cardiology consultants; ACC/AHA antibiotic table
- HACEK endocarditis: Ceftriaxone or ampicillin/sulbactam 4 weeks or ciprofloxacin (ampicillin/ceftriaxone allergy) for 6 weeks

Indications for surgery[10]: **Class I**: heart failure, dehiscence of prosthetic valve, increasing obstruction or insufficiency of the infected prosthetic valve, paravalvular abscess. **Class IIa**: persistent bacteremia or recurrent emboli in setting of appropriate antimicrobial therapy, relapsed infection following therapy.

- Fungal prosthetic valve endocarditis will require surgery plus long-term antifungal therapy.
- Anticoagulation: Switch from warfarin to heparin given possibility of urgent surgery, discontinue aspirin. Discontinue heparin if focal neurologic symptoms develop and image brain
- **Outcomes:**[22] 60% overall 10-year survival, 20% need repeat operation
- **Predictors of worse outcome:**[22] With surgery for PVE
- Early mortality: Older age, female, longer bypass times, emergency surgery, Staph etiology, positive intraoperative culture, severity of preoperative congestive heart failure
- Late mortality: Older age, male, decreased ejection fraction, fungal etiology, extent of infection, and complexity of operative procedure
- **Complications:**[22] Similar to native valve endocarditis
- One series reported a 36% incidence of myocardial abscess and a 63% incidence of paravalvular abscess with prosthetic valve endocarditis. **Relapse rate:**[1] 10% to 15%

MARANTIC ENDOCARDITIS[23–25]

- Libman-Sacks: Patients with systemic lupus erythematosus: Most commonly involves mitral valve
- Increased prevalence in lupus patients with positive anticardiolipin and/or lupus anticoagulant antibodies
- Suggestion of predisposition to bacterial endocarditis from valvular damage and need for antibiotic prophylaxis
- Lack of controlled trials to guide management
- Case reports of valve replacement
- No objective data demonstrating altered course with steroids

- Anticoagulation recommended for patients with valvulopathy and thromboembolic event
- No recommendation for primary prevention anticoagulation at this time
- Underlying neoplasm:[25] Anticoagulation recommended for nonbacterial thrombotic endocarditis and systemic or pulmonary emboli
- Anticoagulation also recommended for patients with disseminated cancer or debilitating disease and marantic vegetations on echo[25]

INDICATIONS FOR ENDOCARDITIS PROPHYLAXIS AND ANTIBIOTIC RECOMMENDATIONS[26]

- Prosthetic heart valve
- Prosthetic material used for valve repair
- History of prior infectious endocarditis
- Patients with cardiac transplant valvulopathy
- Cyanotic congenital heart disease-unrepaired
- Cyanotic congenital heart diasease—surgically or percutaneously repaired in the first six months following repair
- Surgically or percutaneously repaired congenital heart disease with residual defect that impairs endothelialization process[26]
- Prophylaxis is recommended for dental procedures that will disrupt gingival or periapical tissue or oral mucosa.[26]
- Prophylaxis is no longer indicated for gastrointestinal or genitourinary procedures.[24]

REFERENCES

1. Mylonakis E, Calderwood SB. Infective endocarditis in adults. *N Engl J Med*. 2001;345:1318–1330.
2. Hoen B, Epidemiology and antibiotic treatment of infective endocarditis: an update. *Heart*. 92:1694–1700, 2006.
3. Crawford MH, Durack DT. Clinical presentation of infective endocarditis. *Cardiology Clinics*. 21:159–166, 2003.
4. Baddour LM, et al. Infective endocarditis. *Circulation*. 111:394–434, 2005.
5. Li JS, Sexton DJ, Mick N, et al. Proposed modifications to the Duke criteria for the diagnosis of infective endocarditis. *Clin Infect Dis*. 2000;30:633–638.
6. Moreillon P, Que Y, Infective endocarditis. *Lancet*. 363:139–149, 2004.
7. Erbel R, Rohmann S, Drexler M, et al. Improved diagnostic value of echocardiography in patients with infective endocarditis by transesophageal approach. A prospective study. *Eur Heart J*. 1988;9:43–53.
8. Shively BK, Gurule FT, Roldan CA, et al. Diagnostic value of transesophageal compared with transthoracic echocardiography in infective endocarditis. *J Am Coll Cardiol*. 1991;18:391–397.

9. Fowler VG, Li J, Corey GR, et al. Role of echocardiography in evaluation of patients with *Staphylococcus aureus* bacteremia: Experience in 103 patients. *J Am Coll Cardiol.* 1997;30:1072–1078.

10. Bonow RO, et al. ACC/AHA 2006 Guidelines for the management of patients with valvular heart disease. *Am J Cardiol.* 48:1–148, 2006.

11. Andrews MM, von Reyn CF. Patient selection criteria and management guidelines for outpatient parenteral antibiotic therapy for native valve infective endocarditis. *Clin Infect Dis.* 2001;33:203–209.

12. Hasbun R, Vikram HR, Barakat LA, et al. Complicated left-sided native valve endocarditis in adults. *JAMA.* 2003;289:1933–1940, 2003.

13. Moss R, Munt B. Injection drug use and right sided endocarditis. *Heart.* 2003;89:577–581.

14. Vikram HR, Buenconsejo J, Hasbun R, et al. Impact of valve surgery on 6-month mortality in adults with complicated, left-sided native valve endocarditis: A propensity analysis. *JAMA.* 2003;290:3207–3214.

15. Chu VH, Cabell CH, Benjamin DK, et al. Early predictors of in-hospital death in infective endocarditis. *Circulation.* 2004;109:1745–1749.

16. Habib G. Management of infective endocarditis. *Heart.* 2006;92: 124–130.

17. Sexton DJ, Spelman D. Current best practices and guidelines. *Cardiol Clin.* 2003;21:273–282.

18. Chua JD, Wilkoff BL, Lee I, et al. Diagnosis and management of infections involving implantable electrophysiologic cardiac devices. *Ann Intern Med.* 2000;133:604–608.

19. Karchmer AW, Longworth DL. Infections of intracardiac devices. *Cardiol Clin.* 2003;21:253–271.

20. Darouiche RO. Treatment of infections associated with surgical implants. *N Engl J Med.* 2004;350:1422–1429.

21. Cacoub P, Leprince P, Nataf P, et al. Pacemaker infective endocarditis. *Am J Cardiol* 82:480–484, 1998.

22. Mahesh B, Angelini G, Caputo M, et al. Prosthetic valve endocarditis. *Ann Thorac Surg.* 2005;80:1151–1158.

23. Gonzalez-Juanatey C, Gonzalez-Gay MA. Libman-Sacks endocarditis and primary antiphospholipid syndrome. *J Heart Valve Dis.* 2005;14:700–702.

24. Lockshin M, Tenedios F, Petri M, et al. Cardiac disease in the antiphospholipid syndrome: Recommendations for treatment. Committee consensus report. *Lupus.* 2003;12:518–523.

25. Salem DN, Daudelin DH, Levine HJ, et al. Antithrombotic therapy in valvular heart disease. *Chest.* 2001;119:207–219.

26. Wilson W, et al. Prevention of infective endocarditis: Guidelines from the American Heart Association. *Circulation.* 116:1736–1754, 2007.

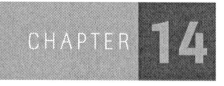

CHAPTER 14

Pericardial Disease

TODD L. KIEFER AND RANDALL VAGELOS

ACUTE PERICARDITIS[1,2]

* **Etiologies**: Idiopathic, viral, tuberculosis (TB), coccidiomycosis, uremia, collagen vascular diseases, neoplasm, trauma, post-myocardial infarction—two types: 1 to 3 days post-transmural infarct and weeks to months postinfarction (Dressler syndrome), prior external beam radiation, HIV
* **Clinical presentation**: Substernal chest pain, pleuritic in nature, +/− radiation to left arm, often radiates to trapezius, pain diminished with sitting up and leaning forward, pain exacerbated with lying supine
  ○ Patient may provide history of fever or recent viral illness
* **Differential diagnosis**: Myocardial infarction, pulmonary embolism, aortic dissection, pneumothorax, pleurisy, costochondritis, gastroesophageal reflux
* **Physical exam**: Triphasic (ventricular systole, early diastole, and atrial contraction) friction rub in 85% of patients, radiates from left lower sternal border to apex, exam often fluctuates
* **Electrocardiogram (ECG)**: Diffuse ST segment elevation with the exception of leads avR and V1

FOUR STAGES OF ECG ABNORMALITIES[1]
1. Diffuse concave S-T elevation and P-R depression
2. Normalization S-T and P-R segments
3. Diffuse T wave inversions
4. Normalization of T waves

* **Laboratory evaluation**: +/− Elevated white blood cell count with lymphocyte predominance, elevated ESR suggests TB or autoimmune etiology, may see minimal troponin elevation (greater elevation suggests

223

myocardial infarction or myocarditis), blood cultures if fever and elevated WBC, pericardial fluid culture if purulent pericarditis is suspected and pericardiocentesis is performed

- **Echocardiography:** Usually normal, may see pericardial effusion
- **Treatment:** Nonsteroidal anti-inflammatory drugs—ibuprofen 600 to 800 mg p.o. tid for 2 weeks
- Prednisone taper over weeks to a month if no improvement with ibuprofen
- Consider evaluation for underlying etiology if recurrent
- Colchicine (COPE Trial):[3] One hundred twenty patients with first episode pericarditis from connective tissue disease, postpericardiotomy, or idiopathic etiology were randomized to aspirin+colchicine versus aspirin alone, and the aspirin+colchicine treatment arm resulted in significantly decreased symptoms at 3 days and recurrent symptoms at 18 months.
- **Predictors of worse outcome:**[1] Temperature $>38°C$, symptoms of several weeks duration in an immunosuppressed patient, traumatic etiology, development of pericarditis while on oral anticoagulation, large effusion greater than 20 mm, evidence of purulent pericarditis without antibiotic treatment >24 hours, postradiation pericarditis often progresses to effusive/constrictive pericarditis
- **Complications:** Enlarging effusion progressing to cardiac tamponade, development of chronic constrictive pericarditis

PERICARDIAL EFFUSION[1,2]

- **Etiologies:** Neoplasm (lung, breast, lymphoma, melanoma), pericarditis, postradiation therapy, trauma, infection (bacterial, fungal, HIV, mycobacterium), uremia, collagen vascular disease, hypothyroidism
- **Cardiac tamponade:** Pericardium exquisitely sensitive to fluctuations in volume over time and will not hemodynamically tolerate rapid accumulation of fluid
- Right heart low-pressure system which is susceptible to compression
- **Clinical presentation:** $+/-$ Chest pain, dyspnea
- **Physical exam:** Tachycardic, jugular venous distinction, decreased heart sounds, paradoxical pulse: >10 mm Hg decrease in systolic arterial pressure with inspiration (can have absent brachial or radial pulse on palpation with inspiration)
- **ECG:** Low voltage, electrical alternans (beat to beat variation in voltage)
- **Invasive hemodynamic data:**[4] Characteristic fall in aortic pressure with inspiration and right atrial pressure tracing pattern with steep x-descent and lack of y-descent
- **Echocardiography:**[1] Right atrial collapse with expiration (sensitive)
  ○ Right ventricular collapse greater than one third of diastole (specific)

- Mitral inflow velocity: With inspiration mitral valve inflow velocity decreases and tricuspid valve inflow velocity increases

  ○ **Treatment:** If tamponade physiology is present administer IV fluids to temporize until pericardiocentesis is performed.

- Use caution with intubation and initiation of mechanical ventilation as positive end-expiratory pressure may induce cardiovascular collapse from further decrease in preload.

PERICARDIAL CONSTRICTION[4-8]

- **Etiologies:** Postpericarditis, postradiation therapy, postcardiac surgery, TB pericarditis
- **Clinical presentation:** Consistent with low cardiac output state manifested by decreased exercise tolerance, cardiac cachexia/wasting, ascites, edema
- **Physical examination:** Jugular venous distention with rapid x and y descent

    Kussmaul's sign: Lack of fall or increase in jugular venous distention (RA pressure) with inspiration due to pericardial limitation preventing transmission of intrathoracic pressure variation to the cardiac chambers

    Pericardial knock: High-pitched, early diastolic sound due to sudden cessation of right ventricular filling from rigid pericardium

- **Laboratory evaluation:** Transaminitis ("cardiac cirrhosis"), BNP <200 usually
- **ECG:** P waves with evidence of intra-atrial conduction delay
- **Chest radiograph:** Globular heart, calcified pericardium, pleural effusions, rarely pulmonary edema
- **Imaging:** Transthoracic echocardiography, transesophageal echocardiography (increased sensitivity compared with transthoracic), computed tomography scan, magnetic resonance imaging—pericardium greater than 2 mm supports diagnosis; echocardiographic evidence of marked respiratory variation of greater than 25% in the mitral inflow E wave velocity (decreases with inspiration and increases with expiration)[1]
- Echocardiographic evidence of marked respiratory variation of greater than 25% in the mitral inflow E wave velocity (decreases with inspiration and increases with expiration)
- Clinical pericardial constriction can occur without evidence of calcification or thickening on imaging.
- **Hemodynamic evaluation:**[7-8] Equalization of diastolic pressure in all four cardiac chambers with the pericardial pressure due to the rigid pericardium

  ○ Hemodynamic data to support a diagnosis of constriction:[7,8]

    - LV/RV interdependence
    - LVEDP-RVEDP <5 mm Hg

- Pulmonary artery systolic pressure < 55 mm Hg
- RVEDP/RVSP > 1/3
- Inspiratory decrease in right atrial pressure < 5 mm Hg
- LV rapid filling wave > 7 mm Hg
- PCWP/LV respiratory gradients > 5 mm Hg

- "Dip and plateau" or "square root sign" waveform of ventricular diastolic pressure due to limitation of rapid early diastolic filling from the rigid pericardium
- Simultaneous left and right heart catheterization demonstrates ventricular interdependence (discordance) with increased right ventricular and decreased left ventricular systolic pressure during inspiration.
- **Treatment:** Pericardiectomy (mortality 6%–12% in various series)

REFERENCES

1. Little WC, Freeman GL. Pericardial disease. *Circulation.* 2006;113: 1622–1632.
2. LeWinter MM, Kabbani S. Pericardial diseases. In: Zipes DP, Libby P, Bonow RO, Braunwald E, eds. *Braunwald's Heart Disease: A Textbook of Cardiovascular Medicine,* 7th ed. Philadelphia: Elsevier Saunders; 2005:1757–1779.
3. Imazio M, et al. Colchicine in addition to conventional therapy for acute pericarditis: results of the colchicine for acute pericarditis (COPE) trial. *Circ.* 112:2012–2016, 2005.
4. Sharkey SW. Beyond the wedge: Clinical physiology and the Swan-Ganz catheter. *Am J Med.* 1987;83:111–122.
5. Hancock EW. Differential diagnosis of restrictive cardiomyopathy and constrictive pericarditis. *Heart.* 2001;86:343–349.
6. Nishimura RA. Constrictive pericarditis in the modern era: A diagnostic dilemma. *Heart.* 2001;86:619–623.
7. Talreja DR, et al. Constrictive pericarditis in the modern era: Novel criteria for diagnosis in the catheterization laboratory. *Jrnl. of Am Coll Cardio.* 51:315–319, 2008.
8. Higano ST, et al. Hemodynamic Rounds Series II: Hemodynamics of constrictive physiology: Influence of respiratory dynamics on ventricular pressures. *Cath. Cardio. Interven.* 46:473–486, 1999.

Central Vascular Access Techniques

IAN BROWN

ASEPTIC PROCEDURES

When performing elective central venipuncture, the provider must follow sterile procedures. Once the skin is grossly clean, scrub a wide area with 2% chlorhexidine for 30 to 60 seconds. Chlorhexidine is preferred over povidone-iodine (Betadine) or alcohol because it reduces catheter-related infection.[1,2] The provider should wash hands with antibacterial soap and water or an alcohol-based waterless product.[3,4] For elective central venous catheter (CVC) placement, the provider should use surgical cap, gown, sterile gloves, mask with face shield, and full-body drape.[5] Scheduled line changes and reducing the number of lumens of a catheter are not useful for preventing infection.[1,6]

Tips
* Have all instruments, kits, and tubes ready at bedside, such that they can be opened in sterile fashion if needed.

THE SELDINGER TECHNIQUE

See Table A-1.

PREPARE

Most hospitals stock prepared kits containing the basic required equipment for placement of a central venous catheter (CVC) except for sterile gloves, saline flushes, and needleless saline-lock hubs.

Equipment Needed
* Preparation and drape: chlorhexidine (2% solution with applicator), full-body fenestrated drape, sterile gloves, gown, mask, and surgical cap

TABLE A-1	General overview of Seldinger Technique	

General Indications	Relative Contraindications	General Risks
Emergency access	Distorted anatomy	Arterial puncture
Inadequate peripheral IV sites	Overlying lesions (e.g., infection, burn, abrasion)	Hematoma
		Air embolism
Extended need for IV access	Risks for sclerosis or thrombosis (e.g., prior long-term cannulation, radiation therapy)	Infection
Frequent blood draws		Nerve injury
Special procedures (e.g., PA catheter, CVP monitoring, transvenous pacemaker)	Proximal vascular injury	Pain
	Severe coagulopathy	Aberrant placement
	Uncooperative patient	Arrhythmia
	Inexperienced provider	Failure of procedure
		Vessel thrombosis
		Arteriovenous fistula

PA, pulmonary artery; CVP, central venous pressure.

- Anesthetic: 1% lidocaine, 5-mL syringe, and 26-gauge needle
- Placement: needle capable of passing guidewire, 10-mL syringe, guidewire, 11-blade scalpel, skin dilator, and catheter of desired size
- Flushing: saline flushes and saline-lock hubs
- Securing the catheter: needle driver, 4-0 or larger nonabsorbable suture material or stapler, suture scissors, and transparent dressing
- Other: antibiotic ointment, gauze pads, and IV tubing

PROCEDURE

- Preparation and drape: use aseptic technique
- Anesthetic: in conscious patients apply lidocaine. Superficially, use a skin wheal. Anesthetize deeper layers including clavicular periosteum if subclavian vein is used.
- Catheter placement (see Figure A-1): While applying negative pressure (i.e., pulling back on syringe plunger) advance needle into vessel (A) until flash of blood in the syringe. Pass the guidewire through the needle (B) into the vessel. Remove the needle (C) while the guidewire remains. Placing the flat edge of an 11-blade scalpel parallel to the wire (D), push down to incise the skin. Depending on the kit used, dilation is either performed by a catheter-over-dilator method (as with a Cordis introducer sheath kit),

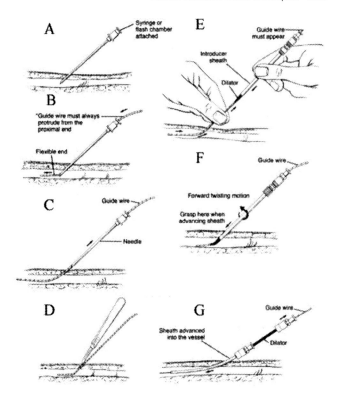

FIGURE A-1 Catheter placement in the Seldinger Technique.[9]

or a separate dilator and catheter. The combined equipment is depicted in Figure A-1. The catheter-over-dilator is threaded onto the guidewire (E). With a firm twisting motion, the dilator and catheter are advanced into the vein (F). Then the dilator is removed with the catheter remaining in the vessel (G). (If a separate dilator is used, after dilation, the dilator is removed while the wire remains. Then place the catheter over the wire into the vessel.) Advance the catheter such that the tip is in the desired position, usually in the vena cava near the right atrium. Remove the wire. *Never let go of the wire as long as it is in the patient.*

- Flush – Perform phlebotomy as needed. Attach saline-lock hub. Attach flush-syringe and *pull back* and confirm good blood flow into syringe. Flush with 10 mL of saline.
- Secure the catheter to the skin with sutures or staples. Depending on the kit used, there is often a butterfly clip and a locking cap that can be used for securing the catheter. Clean, dry, and cover with antibiotic ointment and transparent dressing.

TIPS

- Watch the *New England Journal of Medicine* procedure video on CVC.[7]
- Always order postprocedure chest radiograph after upper body CVC insertion. Specifically review for pneumothorax, hemothorax, and line position.
- If unsure whether catheter is in vein or artery, consider color and pressure of blood. If readily available, check arterial blood gas (ABG) or use pressure transducer. Never dilate the vessel if the wire may be in the artery.
- If using an upper extremity site, prepare both the neck and ipsilateral chest for all jugular and subclavian approaches.
- Always aspirate before injection of an anesthetic.
- Multiple sticks increase likelihood of complications.
- If multiple sticks are used, be sure to flush, or replace, needle after each stick (lidocaine can be used).
- When treating severe sepsis, consider placement of CVC capable of measuring central venous oxygen saturation for use in early goal-directed therapy.[8]

Infraclavicular Approach to the Subclavian Vein
See Table A-2.

Pros: Low rate of infection. Easily identifiable landmarks. Maximizes patient mobility.

Cons: Higher rate of pneumothorax. Noncompressible vessels. Painful.

Position: The patient should be supine to 15-degree Trendelenburg's position, as tolerated, to decrease chance of air embolism. The head should face forward. A small rolled towel can be placed between the scapulae. The right side is preferred[9] because of a lower pleural dome and avoidance of the thoracic duct, except when placing an introducer sheath for procedures (e.g., transvenous pacing or PA catheter placement).

TABLE A-2	The infraclavicular (IC) approach to the subclavian vein	
Specific Indications	Relative Contraindications	Specific Risks

Routine use of CVC
Special procedures
  CVP monitoring
  Temporary pacemaker
Emergency venous access
	Chest wall deformities
	Contralateral pneumothorax
	Enlarged lung fields (e.g., COPD, positive pressure ventilation)
	Hypoxemia
	Coagulopathy/anticoagulation
	Concurrent CPR
	Hemodialysis access
	Ipsilateral pacemaker or ICD
		Pneumothorax
		Hemothorax
		Arterial puncture of noncompressible artery
		Vessel thrombosis
		Brachial plexus injury

ICD, implantable cardioverter defibrillator.

Procedure: Identify and palpate the landmarks—clavicle and sternal notch (Figure A-2). Prepare and drape the patient. In the conscious patient, apply lidocaine, including to the periosteum of the clavicle at point of intersection.

A preferred method[9] is to enter the skin just caudal to the middle of the clavicle. Advance the needle *toward the sternal notch* until it hits the clavicle at the junction of the medial two thirds. While maintaining negative pressure, gently "walk" the needle down the clavicle until it passes directly beneath it. Advance slowly with the needle *horizontal to the plane of the patient*. Blood "flash" is often obtained at a depth of 1 to 2 inches. If the first approach does not yield blood, pull back to skin, fan the needle cephalad, and reinsert. Keeping the needle bevel pointing caudal, pass the guidewire and place catheter as described above.

NOTES

- A straight-tip guidewire is best when entering a straight vessel.
- Needle insertion at the medial aspect of the delta-pectoral groove (at the anterior clavicular tubercle at the junction of the lateral two thirds of the clavicle), may make a technically easier procedure than does midclavicle insertion, but increases the risk of complications including pneumothorax, arterial puncture, and brachial plexus injury.[9,10]
- Don't be afraid to hit the clavicle; the attached vein is directly beneath it. Going too deep increases risk of arterial puncture, brachial plexus injury, or pneumothorax.
- Place the provider's nondominant index finger on the sternal notch (and thumb on clavicle) and aim underneath the index finger, staying horizontal to the plane of the patient. Alternatively, place a fingerprint of blood or povidone-iodine on the drape as a landmark.

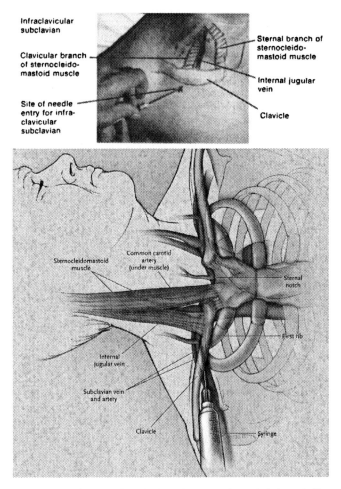

FIGURE A-2 Anatomy for infraclavicular approach to subclavian vein.[34]

Central Approach to the Internal Jugular (IJ) Vein

See Table A-3.

Pros: Low risk of pneumothorax. Good landmarks. Common.

Cons: Difficult in obese patients. Interferes with patient neck movement. Interferes with intubation. Slower than IC. Higher infection rate than IC.

Position: The patient should be supine to 30-degree Trendelenburg's position, as tolerated. The head should face approximately 45 degrees away from the procedure site. If the patient is awake, humming or Valsalva is helpful to engorge the jugular system.[11] The right side has a more direct path to the superior vena cava and avoids the thoracic duct; thus, it is preferred, particularly if placing a Cordis introducer sheath for transvenous pacing.

Procedure: *Ultrasound guidance techniques* are superior to landmark techniques alone, particularly in IJ placement. Ultrasound decreases time of placement, increases chances of successful placement, and reduces mechanical complications.[12-18] It is the method of choice for nonemergent CVC when training and equipment permits.[1,12] Ultrasound should be used in conjunction with the landmark technique as described below.

Identify and palpate the landmarks: The clavicle, the sternocleidomastoid muscle, and the carotid artery. Prepare and drape the patient. The IJ courses down the middle of the triangle formed by the two straps of the sternocleidomastoid muscle heading toward the clavicle (Figure A-3A and B). Because the IJ lies just lateral to the carotid artery, placing fingers from the provider's nondominant hand along the carotid maintains identification of landmarks and decreases chances of arterial puncture.

Apply a wheal of lidocaine at the apex of the cephalad end of the triangle formed by the sternocleidomastoid muscle. Aim at the ipsilateral nipple, while keeping the needle at a 20-degree angle above the plane of the body. While maintaining negative pressure, puncture at this place. Depending on body habitus, expect blood at about 0.5-inch depth. If the vessel is not

TABLE A-3	Central approach to the internal jugular (IJ) vein	
Specific Indications	**Relative Contraindications**	**Specific Risks**
Subclavian vein not accessible	Contralateral pneumothorax	Carotid puncture
Routine use of CVC	Contralateral subclavian attempt	Pneumothorax
Special procedures (e.g., CVP monitoring, transvenous pacemaker)	Obese neck	Hemothorax
	Coagulopathy/anticoagulation	Tracheal perforation
	Concurrent intubation	
	Neck trauma	

(A)

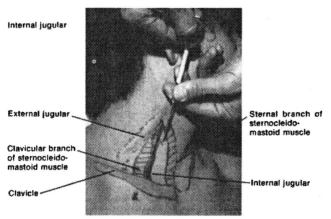

(B)

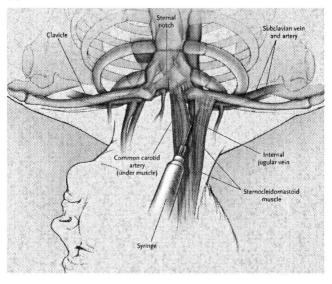

FIGURE A.3, A&B Anatomy for internal jugular (IJ) vein.[6,34]

successfully cannulated, pull back to the skin and fan the needle to a point more medial. Some physicians prefer to start with a 22-gauge "finder needle" attached to a 5-mL syringe to identify the IJ and then use this as a guide for the larger needle through which the wire can be passed as described above.

NOTES

* The right side of the neck is generally easier for right-hand–dominant physicians.
* If the carotid artery is punctured, simply hold pressure with the nondominant hand and continue the procedure.
* The finder needle can be used for lidocaine injection.
* If using a finder needle, the provider can place the procedure needle parallel to the finder needle, or when removing the finder needle, drip a thin line of blood to mark the course of the IJ.

The Femoral Vein

See Table A-4.

Pros: Good landmarks. Quick to place. Easy to apply pressure if artery is punctured.

Cons: Risk of infection and thrombosis. CPR can cause femoral vein pulsation.

Position: The patient should be in supine position. If the physician is right-hand dominant, the patient's right side is usually a technically easier approach.

Procedure: Identify and palpate landmarks. Prepare and drape patient. Place the provider's nondominant hand over the femoral artery pulsation just distal to the inguinal crease. The femoral vein is directly medial to the artery. Apply lidocaine to the conscious patient. Enter the skin at approximately

TABLE A-4	**Femoral vein**	
Specific Indications	Relative Contraindications	Specific Risks
Emergency venous access	Ambulatory patient	Infection
Coagulopathy	Grossly contaminated groin area	Thrombosis
Neck trauma	Penetrating abdominal trauma	Bowel perforation
	No palpable femoral pulse	Bladder perforation
	Known lower extremity deep venous thrombosis (DVT)	

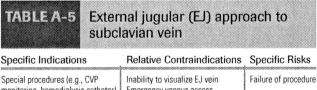

TABLE A-5 External jugular (EJ) approach to subclavian vein

Specific Indications	Relative Contraindications	Specific Risks
Special procedures (e.g., CVP monitoring, hemodialysis catheter)	Inability to visualize EJ vein	Failure of procedure
	Emergency venous access	
Unclear length of stay	Introducer sheath needed	
Pain- or risk-averse patient	Inexperienced provider	

a 45-degree angle. Advance the needle, with negative pressure, until a dark blood flash is returned. Insert catheter via the Seldinger technique.

Pros: The complication rate of an EJ is almost zero; compare to ~13% complication rate for IJ, including very serious complications.[19] For an experienced physician who can visualize the EJ, the excellent risk profile may make the EJ an ideal line for the critically ill patient for whom a complication may be life threatening.[20] An EJ peripheral line can later be converted to a CVC line, if needed. No pain from deep puncture.

Cons: Extra time required for inexperienced physicians to manipulate the wire intrathoracically. Uncommon. The rate of successful EJ placement is only ~76%, compared to ~91% for IJs.[19]

Position: The patient should be supine to 30-degree Trendelenburg's position, as tolerated. The head should face approximately 45 degrees away from the procedure site. If the patient is awake, humming or Valsalva is helpful to engorge the jugular system.[11]

Procedure: In one version of this procedure, an 18-gauge angiocatheter can be placed in the EJ as a peripheral line using sterile precautions. Later, if central venous access is indicated, the line can be converted into a CVC. The site is sterilized, and the IV tubing and saline-lock are removed. A "J" tipped wire[21] is passed via the angiocatheter until an intrathoracic position is presumed (the length of the guidewire must extend past the clavicle). The angiocatheter is then removed. A standard CVC can be passed over the wire via the Seldinger technique.

Supraclavicular Approach to the Subclavian Vein
See Table A-6.

Pros: No need to stop CPR or intubation.[9] Only possible CVC for sitting patient.

Cons: Uncommon. Poor landmarks.

Position: The patient can be in any position from sitting up to 30-degree Trendelenburg's position, as tolerated.

TABLE A-6	The supraclavicular (Super C) approach to the subclavian vein	
Specific Indications	**Relative Contraindications**	**Specific Risks**
Inability to lie supine	Inexperienced provider	Pneumothorax
CPR		Hemothorax

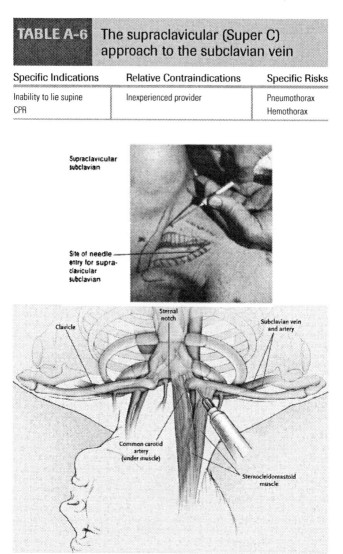

FIGURE A.4 Anatomy for supraclavicular approach to subclavian vein.[34]

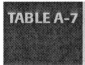

TABLE A-7 Comparison of complication incidence by CVC method; Ease of use in code situation

	IC	IJ	Femoral	EJ	Super C
Unsuccessful placement[25–28]	6%–26%	5%–25%	15%	4%–24%	5%
Mechanical complications[6,25,26]					
Arterial puncture	3%–5%	5%–9%	5%–9%	0%	1%
Hematoma	1%–2%	0%–2%	4%	0%	1%–2%[a]
Pneumothorax	2%–3%	0%	0%	0%	1%
Infection[22,27,29–31]	2–4/1,000 d	8/1,000 d	16–20/1,000 d	0–2/1,000 d	2–4/1,000 d[a]
Thrombosis[27,29,32,33]	0%–15%	0%–40%	21%–25%	0%	0%–15%[a]
Ease of use in code situation	+	−	++	− −	++

[a]Most articles that give complication rate for subclavian vein cannulation do not delineate approach. Data given are for all subclavian.

Procedure: Identify and palpate landmarks. Prepare and drape the patient. The needle is inserted above and behind the medial clavicle (Figure A-4). The syringe bisects the angle formed by the clavicle and the sternal head of the sternocleidomastoid muscle. Aim just caudal to the contralateral nipple. While pulling back on the syringe plunger, insert the needle initially horizontal to the body. If no blood is returned, withdraw the needle to the surface and tilt it such that it is aiming slightly posterior. Cannulation of the bulb where the subclavian vein meets the internal jugular is usually achieved when the syringe is at 15 to 20 degrees above the plane of the body.

COMPLICATIONS OF CVC

Methods for decreasing complications include maximizing physician experience, minimizing catheter indwelling time, using maximum sterile precautions, and choosing a clinically appropriate line with minimal complications (Table A-7). *Antibiotic-impregnated catheters* have been shown to decrease CVC colonization and catheter-related infections.[1,6,22–24] Please refer to the footnoted references for details on reducing complications.[1,6]

REFERENCES

1. O'Grady NP, Alexander M, Dellinger EP, et al. Guidelines for the prevention of intravascular catheter-related infections. *Infect Control Hosp Epidemiol.* 2002;23:759–769.
2. Maki DG, Alvarado CJ, Ringer M. Prospective randomised trial of povidone-iodine, alcohol, and chlorhexidine for prevention of infection associated with central venous and arterial catheters. *Lancet.* 1991;338: 339–343.
3. Larson EL. APIC guideline for handwashing and hand antisepsis in health care settings. *Am J Infect Control.* 1995;23:251–269.
4. Mimoz O, Pieroni L, Lawrence C, et al. Prospective, randomized trial of two antiseptic solutions for prevention of central venous or arterial catheter colonization and infection in intensive care unit patients. *Crit Care Med.* 1996;24:1818–1823.
5. Raad I, Hohn DC, Gilbreath BJ, et al. Prevention of central venous catheter-related infections by using maximal sterile barrier precautions during insertion. *Infect Control Hosp Epidemiol.* 1994;15:231–238.
6. McGee DC, Gould MK. Preventing complications of central venous catheterization. *N Engl J Med.* 2003;348:1123–1133.
7. Graham AS, Ozment C, Tegtmeyer K, et al. Central venous catheterization. *N Engl J Med.* 2007. Available at: http://content.nejm.org/cgi/content/short/356/21/e21/.
8. Rivers E, Nguyen B, Havstad S, et al., for the Early Goal-Directed Therapy Collaborative Group. Early goal-directed therapy in the treatment of severe sepsis and septic shock. *N Engl J Med.* 2001;345:1368–1377.
9. Mickiewicz M, Dronen S, Younger J. Central venous catheterization and central venous pressure monitoring. In: Roberts J, Hedges J, eds. *Roberts: Clinical Procedures in Emergency Medicine.* 4th ed. Philadelphia: WB Saunders; 2004.
10. Simon RR. A new technique for subclavian puncture. *JACEP.* 1978;7:417.
11. Lewin MR, Stein J, Wang R, et al. Humming is as effective as Valsalva's maneuver and Trendelenburg's position for ultrasonographic visualization of the jugular venous system and common femoral veins. *Ann Emerg Med.* 2007.
12. Guidance on the use of ultrasound locating devices for placing central venous catheters. In: *Technology Appraisals.* 49th ed. London: National Institute for Clinical Excellence (NICE); 2002.
13. Teichgraber U, Benter T, Gebel M, et al. A sonographically guided technique for central venous access. *AJR Am J Roentgenol.* 1997;169: 731–733.
14. Bailey PL, Whitaker EE, Palmer LS, et al. The accuracy of the central landmark used for central venous catheterization of the internal jugular vein. *Anesth Analg.* 2006;102:1327–1332.

15. Randolph AG, Cook DJ, Gonzales CA, et al. Ultrasound guidance for placement of central venous catheters: A meta-analysis of the literature. *Crit Care Med.* 1996;24:2053–2058.
16. Leung J, Duffy M, Finckh A. Real-time ultrasonographically-guided internal jugular vein catheterization in the emergency department increases success rates and reduces complications: A randomized, prospective study. *Ann Emerg Med.* 2006;48:540–547.
17. Hind D, Calvert N, McWilliams R, et al. Ultrasonic locating devices for central venous cannulation: Meta-analysis. *BMJ.* 2003;327:361.
18. Rothschild J. Ultrasound guidance of central venous catheterization. In: Wachter R, ed. *Evidence Report/Technology Assessment No. 43, Making Health Care Safer: A Critical Analysis of Patient Safety Practices.* Rockville, MD: Agency for Healthcare Research and Quality; 2001.
19. Belani K, Buckley J, Gordon J, et al. Percutaneous cervical central venous line placement: A comparison of the internal and external jugular vein routes. *Anesth Analg.* 1980;59:40–44.
20. Byth PL. Evaluation of the technique of central venous catheterisation via the external jugular vein using the J-wire. *Anaesth Intensive Care.* 1985;13:131–133.
21. Blitt CD, Wright WA, Petty WC, et al. Central venous catheterization via the external jugular vein. A technique employing the J-WIRE. *JAMA.* 1974;229:817–818.
22. Heard S, Wagle M, Vijayakumar E, et al. Influence of triple-lumen central venous catheters coated with chlorhexidine and silver sulfadiazine on the incidence of catheter-related bacteremia. *Arch Intern Med.* 1998;158:81–87.
23. Raad I, Darouiche R, Dupuis J, et al. Central venous catheters coated with minocycline and rifampin for the prevention of catheter-related colonization and bloodstream infections: A randomized, double-blind trial. *Ann Intern Med.* 1997;127:267–274.
24. Maki DG, Stolz SM, Wheeler S, et al. Prevention of central venous catheter-related bloodstream infection by use of an antiseptic-impregnated catheter: A randomized, controlled trial. *Ann Intern Med.* 1997;127:257–266.
25. Brahos G. Central venous catheterization via the supraclavicular approach. *J Trauma.* 1977;17:872–877.
26. Eisen LA, Narasimhan M, Berger JS, et al. Mechanical complications of central venous catheters. *J Intensive Care Med.* 2006;21:40–46.
27. Cho SK, Shin SW, Do YS, et al. Use of the right external jugular vein as the preferred access site when the right internal jugular vein is not usable. *J Vasc Interv Radiol.* 2006;17:823–829.
28. Sterner S, Plummer DW, Clinton J, et al. A comparison of the supraclavicular approach and the infraclavicular approach for subclavian vein catheterization. *Ann Emerg Med.* 1986;15:421–424.

29. Merrer J, De Jonghe B, Golliot F, et al., for the French Catheter Study Group in Intensive Care. Complications of femoral and subclavian venous catheterization in critically ill patients: A randomized controlled trial. *JAMA*. 2001;286:700–707.

30. McKinley S, Mackenzie A, Finfer S, et al. Incidence and predictors of central venous catheter related infection in intensive care patients. *Anaesth Intensive Care*. 1999;27:164–169.

31. Torok-Both CJ, Jacka MJ, Brindley PG. Best evidence in critical care medicine: Central venous catheterization: The impact of insertion site. *Can J Anaesth*. 2006;53:524–525.

32. Timsit J, Farkas J, Boyer J, et al. Central vein catheter-related thrombosis in intensive care patients: Incidence, risk factors, and relationship with catheter-related sepsis. *Chest*. 1998;114:207–213.

33. Trottier SJ, Veremakis C, O'Brien J, et al. Femoral deep vein thrombosis associated with central venous catheterization: Results from a prospective, randomized trial. *Crit Care Med*. 1995;23:52–59.

34. Knopp R, Dailey RH. Central venous cannulation and pressure monitoring. *JACEP*. 1977;6:358–366.

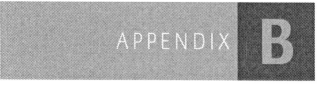

Clinical Pharmacology

KELLY MATSUDA

TABLE B-1 Vasopressors, inotropes, and vasodilators

Drug	Dose	α	β	Dop	CO	PCWP	SVR	BP	HR	ARR	Cautions/clinical effects
Dopamine	1–2 µg/kg/min not recommended	+	+	+++	↑?	?	?	?	?	?	Stimulates dopaminergic DA1 receptors in the renal mesenteric and coronary beds resulting in vasodilation
	2–10 µg/kg/min	++	++	++	↑	?	0	?	↑	↑	Causes NE release from nerve terminals
	10–20 µg/kg/min	+++	++	+	↑	?0	↑	↑	↑	↑	↑ MVO_2
Epinephrine	1–20 µg/min	++	+++	0	↑	↑	↑	↑	↑	↑	May induce tachyarrhythmias
Norepinephrine	1–30 µg/min	+++	++	0	↔/↑	↕	↑	↑	↕	+/−	May induce tachyarrhythmias and myocardial ischemia
Phenylephrine	40–180 µg/min	+++	0	0	↓	?	↑	↑	↓	↑	May cause reflex bradycardia
Vasopressin	0.01–0.04 units/min	0	0	0	↕	↕	↑	↑	↕	↑	Direct stimulation smooth muscle V1 receptors Myocardial ischemia, cardiac dysfunction, arrhythmias reported

	Dose	α	β	Dop	CO	SVR	PCWP	BP	HR	Toxicities
Dobutamine	2–20 μg/kg/min	+	+++	0	↑↑	↓/0	↓/0	↑↑	↑	Tachyarrhythmias
Milrinone	0.375–0.75 μg/kg/min	0	0	0	↑↑	↓	↓	↑	↑	Noncatecholamine, PDI, PI, VD, ARR, adjust dose in renal failure
Nesiritide	0.01 μg/kg/min	0	0	0	↑	↓↓	↓↓	0	0	Hypotension, VD
Nitroglycerin	5–400 μg/min	0	0	0	↑	↓↓	↓	↓↓	↑/0	VD, hypotension, tolerance
Nitroprusside	0.5–2 μg/kg/min	0	0	0	↑	↓↓↓	↓↓↓	↓↓↓	↑	VD, hypotension, reflex tachycardia, caution in renal insufficiency secondary accumulation of thiocyanate and cyanide toxicities

α, alpha agonist; β, beta agonist; Dop, dopaminergic-1 agonist; CO, cardiac output; PCWP, pulmonary capillary wedge pressure; SVR, systemic vascular resistance; BP, blood pressure; HR, heart rate; ARR, arrhythmias; min, minutes; NE, norepinephrine; PDI, phosphodiesterase inhibitor; PI, positive inotrope; VD, vasodilation.

TABLE B-2 Antiarrhythmic medication properties

Drug	Mechanism of Action	Pharmacokinetics	Adverse Effects, Contraindications	Drug Interactions	Dosing by Indication	Comments
Quinidine	Strong vagolytic, anticholinergic properties, Na$^+$ channel blockade	$t_{1/2}$ = 5–9 h	AE: Nausea, vomiting, diarrhea (30%), proarrhythmic, cinchonism HF exacerbations	Warfarin	Afib maintenance: Sulfate 200–400 mg q6h Gluconate 324 mg q8–12h	TR = 6–9 mg/L
Procainamide	Na$^+$ channel blockade	(SA) $t_{1/2}$ = 5–6 h (FA) $t_{1/2}$ = 2–3 h	AE: Decrease dose in renal and liver dysfunction, active metabolite NAPA accumulates, lupuslike syndrome in 30% of patients if >6 months of treatment, hypotension (IV) 30%	—	Afib conversion (IV): 1 g over 30 min, then 2–4 mg/min Afib maintenance: 1–2 g/d in divided doses VT (preserved LVEF >40%): 20 mg/min loading dose infusion until 17 mg/kg, arrhythmia ceases, or QRS widens >50% VT maintenance: 2–4 mg/min	TR = 4–15

Disopyramide	Potent Na⁺ and M₂ blockade, strong negative inotropic effects	$t_{1/2} = 4-8$ h	AE: Anticholinergic side effects: Urinary retention, constipation, tachycardia, dry eyes CI: Glaucoma	—	Afib conversion: 200 mg po q4h (max 800 mg) Maintenance 400–600 mg/d in divided doses	TR = 2–6
Lidocaine	Inactive Na⁺ channel blocker	$t_{1/2} = 1-3$ h	AE: CNS symptoms, periorbital numbness, seizures, confusion, blurry vision, tinnitus CI: Third-degree A-V heart block	—	VT/VF conversion: Pulseless VT/VF or stable VT with LVEF >40%: 1–1.5 mg/kg IVP ×2; 0.5–0.75 mg/kg q3–5 min thereafter max 3 mg/kg VT maintenance: 1–2 mg/min	Dose adjust in patients with liver, renal, or heart failure and in elderly TR = 1.5–5

(continued)

TABLE B-2 (Continued)

Drug	Mechanism of Action	Pharmacokinetics	Adverse Effects, Contraindications	Drug Interactions	Dosing by Indication	Comments
Mexiletine	Inactive Na$^+$ channel blocker	(PM) $t_{1/2}$ = 12–20 h (EM) $t_{1/2}$ = 7–11 h	AE: psychosis, aggravation of underlying conduction disturbances, ventricular arrhythmias CI: Third-degree A-V heart block		VT maintenance: 200–300 mg po q8h	TR = 0.8–2
Propafenone	Na$^+$ and Ca^{2+} channel blocker, β-blocker	(PM) $t_{1/2}$ = 10–25 h (EM) $t_{1/2}$ = 3–7 h	AE: Metallic taste, dizziness CI: HF (causes exacerbation), liver disease, valvular disease (torsade de pointes)	Digoxin ↑ by 70%; warfarin ↑ by 50%	Afib conversion: 600 mg po ×1 Afib maintenance: 150–300 mg po q8–12h	Can use in NYHA class I and II safely
Flecainide	Strong Na$^+$ channel blockade; vagolytic, anticholinergic, and negative inotropic effects	(PM) $t_{1/2}$ = 14–20 h (EM) $t_{1/2}$ = 10–14 h	AE: HF exacerbation, dizziness, tremor, bronchospasm CI: HF (causes exacerbations), CAD, valvular disease, LV hypertrophy, (torsade de pointes)	Digoxin ↑ by 25%	Afib conversion: 300 mg po ×1 Afib maintenance: 50–150 mg q12h	TR = 0.3–2.5

Drug	Mechanism / Pharmacology	Adverse Effects	Interactions	Dosing	Notes
Amiodarone	Na$^+$, K$^+$, Ca^{2+} channel blocker, β-blocker; $t_{1/2}$ = 15–100 d; Inhibits cytochrome P450 (CYP) metabolism CYP2C9, CYP 2D6, CYP3A4; Inhibits glycoprotein in GI tract to increase digoxin bioavailability	AE: Pulmonary fibrosis (3%–17%); hypothyroidism (30%–50%); neurologic toxicity (20%–40%); blue-gray skin (15%); torsade de pointes (<1%); A-V block (14%); hypotension, phlebitis (IV) CI: Iodine hypersensitivity, hyperthyroidism, heart block	Warfarin, digoxin, phenytoin ↑ ≥ 50%	Afib conversion IV: 300 mg IV over 60 min, then 20 mg/kg over 24 h PO: 400 mg tid ×5 to 7 days (8 to 10g) Afib maintenance: 100–200 mg/d Pulseless VT/VF conversion: 300 mg IVP ×1, repeat 150 mg IVP q 3–5 min (ARREST trial), or (ALIVE trial): 5 mg/kg IVP, repeat 2.5 mg/kg Stable VT: 150 mg IVP ×1 over 10 minutes VT/VF maintenance: 1 mg/min × 6 h then 0.5 mg/min (max = 2.2 g/d)	Does not increase mortality in heart failure patients TR = 1–2.5

(continued)

TABLE B-2 *(Continued)*

Drug	Mechanism of Action	Pharmacokinetics	Adverse Effects, Drug Interactions, Contraindications	Dosing by Indication	Comments
Sotalol	Blocks β_1, β_2 receptors, K^+ channels	$t_{1/2} = 10$–20 h	HF exacerbation, bradycardia, wheezing; torsade (3%–8%) within 3 days of initiation; bronchospasm CI: Baseline $QT_c > 440$ ms or CrCL < 40 mL/min in atrial arrhythmias	Not effective for Afib conversion Afib maintenance: CrCL 80 mg bid >60 mL/min 80 mg q36–48h 10–30 mL/min 80 mg >q48h <10 mL/min	Double dose q3d: NTE $QT_c > 440$ ms or CrCL < 20 mL/min Mandatory hospitalization for initiation
Dofetilide	Pure K^+ channel blocker only	$t_{1/2} = 6$–10 h	Torsade de pointes (0.8%–4%); if no real adjustments, dizziness, diarrhea CI: Baseline $QT_c > 440$ ms or CrCL < 20 mL/min DI: 3A4 inhibitors or drugs secreted by kidney: cimetidine, ketoconazole, verapamil, trimethoprim, prochlorperazine, megestrol	Afib conversion: 500 μg po bid if CrCL >60 mL/min 250 mg po bid if CrCL 40–60 mL/min 125 μg po bid if CrCL 20–40 mL/min (efficacy 12% at 1 mo) Afib maintenance: Titrate upward based on QT_c NTE 500 ms or >15% ↑ in QT_c after each dose	Does not increase mortality in HF patients Mandatory hospitalization for initiation ECG after each dose while hospitalized
Ibutilide	Strong K^+ blocker; also Na^+ and β-blocking effects	$t_{1/2} = 3$–6 h	AE: Torsade risk (8%) CI: Receiving concomitant antiarrhythmics or $QT_c > 440$ ms before initiation DI: 3A4 inhibitors or QT-prolonging drugs	Conversion: 1 mg ×1 IV ($\geq$ 60 kg), repeat in 10 min if ineffective (efficacy 47% at 90 min)	Requires ECG monitoring during and after cardioversion

$t_{1/2}$, half-life; AE, adverse effects; TR, therapeutic range; HF, heart failure; CI, contraindications; CrCL, creatinine clearance; Afib, atrial fibrilation; NTE, not to exceed; IV, left ventricular; DI, drug interactions; IV, intravenous; CAD, coronary artery disease; PM, poor metabolizers; EM, extensive metabolizers.

TABLE B-3 Pharmacological rate control with atrial fibrillation: Acute setting (without accessory pathway)

Drug	Mechanism of Action	Pharmacokinetics	Adverse Reactions, Drug Interactions, Contraindications	Dosing	Comments
Esmolol	β₁ blockade	Onset: 5 min $t_{1/2}$ = 9 min	↓BP, ↓HR, HF, HB CI: Asthma DI: Beta agonist	500 μg/kg IV bolus over 1 min Then 25–50 μg/kg/min infusion To maximum 200 μg/kg/min	Beta blocker toxicity use intravenous atropine, pressors (dopamine, dobutamine, epinephrine, isoproterenol, or glucagon bradycardia, and asystole intravenous atropine, pressors (dopamine, dobutamine, epinephrine, isoproterenol, or glucagon and/or temporary ventricular pacing may be initiated
Metoprolol	β₁ blockade	Onset: 5 min $t_{1/2}$ = 3–7 h	↓BP, ↓HR, HF, HB CI: Asthma DI: Beta agonist	2.5–5 mg IV q5min ×3 doses	Beta blocker toxicity use intravenous atropine, pressors (dopamine, dobutamine, epinephrine, isoproterenol, or glucagon bradycardia, and asystole intravenous atropine, pressors (dopamine, dobutamine, epinephrine, isoproterenol, or glucagon and/or temporary ventricular pacing may be initiated

(continued)

TABLE B-3 (Continued)

Drug	Mechanism of Action	Pharmacokinetics	Adverse Reactions, Drug Interactions, Contraindications	Dosing	Comments
Diltiazem	↓S-A and ↓A-V node conduction	Onset 2–7 min $t_{1/2}$ = 4–10 h	HB, ↓BP, ↓HR	0.25 mg/kg IV over 3 min then 5–15 mg/h IV continuous	Ca^{2+} overdose, use IV calcium 1–2 g to reverse hypotension Use intravenous atropine, pressors (dopamine, dobutamine, epinephrine, isoproterenol), or glucagon bradycardia, and asystole intravenous atropine, pressors (dopamine, dobutamine, epinephrine, isoproterenol), or glucagon and/or temporary ventricular pacing may be initiated
Verapamil	↓S-A and ↓A-V node conduction	Onset 3–5 min $t_{1/2}$ = 4–12 h	HB, ↓BP, ↓HR	0.075–0.15 mg/kg IV over 2 min	Ca^{2+} overdose, use IV calcium 1–2 g to reverse hypotension Use intravenous atropine, pressors (dopamine, dobutamine, epinephrine, isoproterenol), or glucagon for bradycardia, asystole, and/or temporary ventricular pacing may be initiated

$t_{1/2}$, half-life; ADR, adverse drug reactions; BP, blood pressure; HR, heart rate; HF, heart failure; HB, heart block; CI, contraindications; DI, drug interactions.
From Fuster V, Ryden LE, Cannom DS, et al. ACC/AHA/ESC guidelines for the management of patients with atrial fibrillation: Executive summary. A report of the American College of Cardiology/American Heart Association Task Force on Practice Guidelines and the European Society of Cardiology Committee for Practice Guidelines. *Circulation.* 2006;114:700–752.

TABLE B-4 Heart rate control without accessory pathway with heart failure

Drug	Mechanism of Action	Pharmacokinetics	Adverse Drug Reactions, Contraindications, Drug Interactions	Dosing	Comments
Digoxin	Negative chromotrope Positive inotrope	Onset: 60 min or longer $t_{1/2}$ = 1.8–2.2 d	ADR: Digitalis toxicity, HB, ↓ HR	10 μg/kg IV loading based on lean body wt. then 0.125–0.25 mg daily IV	Monitor renal function, digoxin will accumulate in renal dysfunction Some subgroup evidence to target dig level <1.2 Symptomatic digoxin toxicity, use Digoxin Immune Fab (Digibind)
Amiodarone	Na^+ channel blockade, beta blockade, Ca^{2+} channel blockade, K^+ channel blockade, and vasodilatory effects	Onset: Days $t_{1/2}$ = 50 d	ADR: ↓BP, HB, pulmonary toxicity, skin discoloration, hypothyroidism, hyperthyroidism, corneal deposits, optic neuropathy, sinus bradycardia DI: Warfarin, digoxin	150 mg over 10 min, then 0.5–1 mg/min	Caution: Concentration for central line administration vs. peripheral line administration (phlebitis)

$t_{1/2}$, half-life; ADR, adverse drug reactions; HB, heart block; HR, heart rate; BP, blood pressure; DI, drug interactions.

TABLE B-5 Heart rate control with accessory pathway

Drug	Mechanism of Action	Pharmacokinetics	Adverse Drug Reactions, Drug Interactions	Dosing	Comments
Amiodarone	Na^+ channel blockade, beta blockade, Ca^{2+} channel blockade, K^+ channel blockade, and vasodilatory effects	Onset: Days $t_{1/2} = 50$ d	ADR: ↓BP, HB, pulmonary toxicity, skin discoloration, hypothyroidism, hyperthyroidism, corneal deposits, optic neuropathy, sinus bradycardia DI: Warfarin, digoxin	150 mg over 10 min, then 0.5–1 mg/min	Caution: Concentration for central line administration vs. peripheral line administration (phlebitis)

$t_{1/2}$, half-life; ADR, adverse drug reactions; BP, blood pressure; HB, heart block; DI, drug interactions.

INDEX